Leadership

Guest Editor

NANCY GIRARD, PhD, RN, FAAN

PERIOPERATIVE NURSING CLINICS

www.periopnursing.theclinics.com

Consulting Editor
NANCY GIRARD, PhD, RN, FAAN

March 2009 • Volume 4 • Number 1

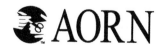

SAUNDERS an imprint of ELSEVIER, Inc.

W.B. SAUNDERS COMPANY
A Division of Elsevier Inc.

1600 John F. Kennedy Boulevard ● Suite 1800 ● Philadelphia, Pennsylvania 19103-2899

http://www.periopnursing.theclinics.com

PERIOPERATIVE NURSING CLINICS Volume 4, Number 1
March 2009 ISSN 1556-7931, ISBN-13: 978-1-4377-0522-5, ISBN-10: 1-4377-0522-7

Editor: Katie Hartner

Photocopying
Single photocopies of single articles may be made for personal use as allowed by national copyright laws. Permission of the Publisher and payment of a fee is required for all other photocopying, including multiple or systematic copying, copying for advertising or promotional purposes, resale, and all forms of document delivery. Special rates are available for educational institutions that wish to make photocopies for non-profit educational classroom use. For information on how to seek permission visit www.elsevier.com/permissions or call: (+44) 1865 843830 (UK)/(+1) 215 239 3804 (USA).

Derivative Works
Subscribers may reproduce tables of contents or prepare lists of articles including abstracts for internal circulation within their institutions. Permission of the Publisher is required for resale or distribution outside the institution. Permission of the Publisher is required for all other derivative works, including compilations and translations (please consult www.elsevier.com/permissions).

Electronic Storage or Usage
Permission of the Publisher is required to store or use electronically any material contained in this journal, including any article or part of an article (please consult www.elsevier.com/permissions). Except as outlined above, no part of this publication may be reproduced, stored in a retrieval system or transmitted in any form or by any means, electronic, mechanical, photocopying, recording or otherwise, without prior written permission of the Publisher.

Notice
No responsibility is assumed by the Publisher for any injury and/or damage to persons or property as a matter of products liability, negligence or otherwise, or from any use or operation of any methods, products, instructions or ideas contained in the material herein. Because of rapid advances in the medical sciences, in particular, independent verification of diagnoses and drug dosages should be made

Although all advertising material is expected to conform to ethical (medical) standards, inclusion in this publication does not constitute a guarantee or endorsement of the quality or value of such product or of the claims made of it by its manufacturer.

The ideas and opinions expressed in *Perioperative Nursing Clinics* do not necessarily reflect those of the Publisher nor the Association of periOperative Registered Nurses (AORN, Inc). Neither the Publisher nor AORN Inc assume any responsibility for any injury and/or damage to persons or property arising out of or related to any use of the material contained in this periodical. The reader is advised to check the appropriate medical literature and the product information currently provided by the manufacturer of each drug to be administered to verify the dosage, the method and duration of administration, or contraindications. It is the responsibility of the treating physician or other health care professional, relying on independent experience and knowledge of the patient, to determine drug dosages and the best treatment for the patient. Mention of any product in this issue should not be construed as endorsement by the contributors, editors, AORN Inc, or the Publisher of the product or manufacturers' claims. The content of this issue has not been peer reviewed by AORN Inc, and AORN Inc makes no representation as to compliance of the content with the AORN Inc standards, recommended practices or guidelines. AORN's endorsement of the publication does not constitute endorsement of any representations or assertions in the content.

Perioperative Nursing Clinics (ISSN 1556-7931) is published quarterly by Elsevier, 360 Park Avenue South, New York, NY 10010. Months of issue are March, June, September and December. Business and Editorial Offices: 1600 John F. Kennedy Blvd., Suite 1800, Philadelphia, PA 19103-2899. Customer Service Office: 11830 Westline Industrial Drive, St. Louis, MO 63146. Periodicals postage paid at New York, NY and at additional mailing offices. Subscription prices are $116.00 per year (domestic individuals), $209.00 per year (domestic institutions), $58.00 per year (domestic students/residents), $116.00 per year (Canadian individuals), $240.00 per year (Canadian institutions), $150 per year (international individuals), $240 per year (international institutions), and $62.00 per year (International and Canadian students/residents). Foreign air speed delivery is included in all Clinics subscription prices. All prices are subject to change without notice. **POSTMASTER:** Send change of address to *Perioperative Nursing Clinics*, Customer Service (orders, claims online, change of address): Elsevier Periodicals Customer Service, 11830 Westline Industrial Drive, St. Louis, MO 63146. Tel: 1-800-654-2452 (U.S. and Canada). Fax: 314-523-5170. E-mail: journalscustomerservice-usa@elsevier.com (for print support); journalsonlinesupport-usa@elsevier.com (for online support).

Reprints. For copies of 100 or more, of articles in this publication, please contact the Commercial Reprints Department, Elsevier Inc., 360 Park Avenue South, New York, NY 10010-1710. Tel. (212) 633-3812; Fax: (212) 462-1935; email: reprints@elsevier.com.

Printed and bound by CPI Group (UK) Ltd, Croydon, CR0 4YY

Transferred to Digital Print 2011

Contributors

CONSULTING EDITOR

NANCY GIRARD, PhD, RN, FAAN
Consultant, Boerne; Clinical Associate
Professor, Acute Nursing Care Department,
University of Texas Health Science Center, San
Antonio, Texas

GUEST EDITOR

NANCY GIRARD, PhD, RN, FAAN
Consultant, Boerne; Clinical Associate
Professor, Acute Nursing Care Department,
University of Texas Health Science Center,
San Antonio, Texas

AUTHORS

CYNTHIA BARRERE, PhD, RN, AHN-BC
Associate Professor of Nursing, Department
of Nursing, Undergraduate Nursing Program,
Quinnipiac University, Hamden, Connecticut

**VICKI D. BATSON, RN, MSN, CNOR,
NEA-BC**
Doctoral Student, The University of Texas
at Austin School of Nursing; Staff Nurse IV,
Operating Room, Seton Medical Center,
Austin, Texas

PATRICIA A. CORNETT, EdD, MS, RN
Principal, Solucion International—Workforce
and Workplace Solutions, Canyon Lake, Texas

NANCY GIRARD, PhD, RN, FAAN
Consultant, Boerne; Clinical Associate
Professor, Acute Nursing Care Department,
University of Texas Health Science Center, San
Antonio, Texas

LYNN KEEGAN, PhD, RN, AHN-BC, FAAN
Director, Holistic Nursing Consultants, Port
Angeles, Washington

DENISE M. KORNIEWICZ, PhD, RN, FAAN
Professor and Senior Associate Dean for
Research, University of Miami, School of
Nursing and Health Studies, Coral Gables,
Florida

GEORGE F. NUSSBAUM, PhD, RN, CNOR
Assistant Professor, Graduate School
of Nursing, Uniformed Services University
of the Health Sciences, Bethesda,
Maryland

JOANNE D. OLIVER, RN, BSN, CNOR
AORN State Council Leadership Chair; and
Co-Chair, Texas State Council; and Chair,
AORN Greater Houston Legislative Committee,
West Houston, Texas

CHRISTINE M. PACINI, PhD, RN
Director, Center for Professional Development,
Research and Innovation, Department of
Nursing Services, University of Michigan
Health System, Ann Arbor, Michigan

MICKEY L. PARSONS, PhD, MHA, RN, FAAN
Associate Professor and Coordinator, Graduate Administration Program, The University of Texas Health Science Center at San Antonio School of Nursing, San Antonio, Texas

CAROL A. REINECK, PhD, MSN, MAEd, RN, FAAN, NEA-BC
Retired, Colonel, U.S. Army; Chair and Associate Professor, Department of Acute Nursing Care; and Amy Shelton and V.H. McNutt Professor in Honor of Nurses of the Armed Forces, The University of Texas Health Science Center at San Antonio School of Nursing, San Antonio, Texas

JEANNE H. SIEGEL, PhD, FNP
Assistant Professor, University of Miami, School of Nursing and Health Studies, Coral Gables, Florida

VICTORIA M. STEELMAN, PhD, RN, CNOR, FAAN
Advanced Practice Nurse, Department of Nursing, The University of Iowa Hospitals and Clinics, Iowa City, Iowa

LINDA H. YODER, RN, MBA, PhD, AOCN, FAAN
Associate Professor; and Luci Baines Johnson Fellow in Nursing; and Director, Nursing Administration and Health Care Systems Management, The University of Texas at Austin School of Nursing, Austin, Texas

Contents

> To accomplish the clinical care, leadership is critical. Leadership helps integrate the efforts of the entire surgical team amid simultaneous pressures to achieve the expectations of the access, quality, and cost triad. Leadership in the context of contemporary perioperative nursing practice can be learned, practiced, and improved. Leadership content does not change; the context in which it is practiced does change. A framework of five exemplary leadership practices is described. The five leadership practices provide a simple and useful framework to guide perioperative nursing leadership. Highlighting the portability of this framework across settings, each practice is briefly illustrated in the markedly contrasting environments of the military and academia, with a recommendation for use in perioperative nursing practice.

> Leadership development resources are plentiful and span all modes of delivery ranging from self-help workbooks to graduate degree-granting programs. The competencies required to fulfill the expectations of the role are many and assorted. Yet, one of the most important areas, establishing a healthy workplace, is rarely included. This paper describes how a manager can empower staff via a healthy workplace intervention while also honing new leadership skills through experiential learning that occurs during all phases of the intervention.

> To ensure the direction of perioperative nursing, one must learn to inform, educate, negotiate, and stimulate others to do the same. This article discusses specifics on each of these items as they relate to perioperative nursing and legislation.

> This article presents variables not commonly considered in presenting leadership theory. Effective leadership requires more than a list of attributes of the leader; it requires the potential leader's ability to understand specific nuances of those expected to follow. In a culturally diverse organization, significant behavioral norms,

part of each individual's cultural heritage, are uniquely present and potentially different in each workplace subordinate. A leader's understanding of these cultural variances can significantly reduce communication mishaps and avoid many nonproductive leadership challenges. The variables discussed are the cultural differences in the concept of time, allowable social and workplace expressiveness, oculesic and kinesetic (paralinguistic) variances, counseling dynamics and forgiveness in the organizational culture, and the groupthink phenomenon.

Nurses today are faced with multiple tasks and institutional demands that require continued change in the clinical environment. Because of concerns raised by national and international studies associated with the cost of health care, patient safety factors, and new regulations associated with reimbursement, nurses at the bedside are being asked to improve patient care outcomes. Therefore, most staff nurses lack the skills associated with evidence-based approaches or data-driven results. In fact, most clinicians must be reeducated about their role within the organization and as an active member in gathering data, participating in clinical research forums, or working with multidisciplinary teams to promote new clinical treatments.

Nurse leaders are essential in all areas of health care. Their visions for health care improvement and ability to inspire others to work to their full potential to realize these visions involve a tremendous amount of work and creativity. To maintain the strength and resilience needed to be successful, nurse leaders must also practice effective stress management strategies that help them remain focused, centered, and calm. Nurse leaders need to understand themselves in body, mind, and spirit to reflect on the balance of these aspects of self within them and determine where they need to focus to rise above the stress by rebalancing their internal and external healing environments.

Educational leadership has forged the nursing profession that exists today. This article briefly reviews the historical beginning of education with Florence Nightingale, and the types of nursing education available today. This article summarizes the leadership characteristics, skills needed, and outcomes desired of educators at the dean, department chair, faculty, and staff development educator level.

The advanced practice nurse has a vital role in the perioperative leadership team. This person through advanced education coupled with clinical expertise has the background to positively influence the quality of patient care, improve staff safety, and implement evidence-based interdisciplinary changes. The discussion herein focuses on the leadership role of the clinical nurse specialist.

This article discusses the influence of nurse manager coaching as a transformational leadership skill and describes an effective process for coaching staff. Although each employee is a unique individual, generational differences that have a direct effect on coaching have been identified. Knowing these differences can assist the nurse manager in using coaching more effectively with these groups. Finally, a primary outcome of coaching is to develop self efficacy of staff. By starting to coach direct reports who have either formal or informal leadership responsibilities, the nurse manager can disseminate a coaching culture within the department as a strategy to foster growth, development, and autonomy at all levels.

Given the current demands of the health care environment, the need for nurses minimally competent in clinical judgment, caring practice, advocacy and moral agency, collaboration, responsiveness to diversity, systems thinking, inquiry, and facilitation of learning is critical in light of ever-increasing contextual complexity and variability of patient needs. The Synergy Model provides an exemplary and relevant framework for clinical practice with the ultimate aim of improving patient outcomes. Tenets of accountability and professionalism are central to the model and, in its entirety, it provides a practical and useful approach for thinking about and redesigning educational products and processes in clinical settings.

Perioperative Nursing Clinics

THE CLINICS ARE NOW AVAILABLE ONLINE!

Access your subscription at:
www.theclinics.com

Foreword

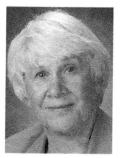

Nancy Girard, PhD, RN, FAAN
Consulting Editor

This issue of *Perioperative Nursing Clinics* focuses on leadership, which is both a tangible and intangible role, and leadership also can be formal or informal. A strong leader is greatly desired, and while many aspire to be leaders, some never rise to the role. The world hunts for leaders; people want strong leaders; and true leaders are everywhere, but they often are not recognized unless the position they hold is a formal one. Good leaders find that people want to follow them. It has been said that it is lonely at the top and formal leaders often have no peers they can confide in or toss ideas around with. While many attempt to teach leadership, and others struggle to learn the skills of leadership, some think one can only be born with leadership ability. There are overlapping characteristics and character traits of good leaders, and the reader will see those depicted in the articles in this issue.

I am sure that each of us remembers leaders that have guided our path or affected our career. I vividly remember one that I will share with you. During my medical-surgical course in nursing school, when I was obtaining my baccalaureate degree, my clinical practicum was with a director of the operating room at a large city hospital. I was to work with this director to learn the perioperative manager role. This occurred four decades ago, so you can determine for yourself how futuristic a leader she was. The director's philosophy was that perioperative nurses should care for the patient during the total surgical experience. Therefore, my assignment was to plan total care for a woman who was scheduled for an open cholecystectomy (the only kind done in those days.)

She had just delivered her sixth child 2 days previously. I was sent to her house to do a preoperative assignment and prepare her for surgery. Among the routine information, I found she was afraid of an anesthesia mask and was breast feeding. We arranged for all aspects of care, including not using anesthesia masks, allowing her to breast feed, and providing an adjoining room, where her husband and new baby could stay while she was recuperating. The patient was hospitalized for 4 days in those days for an open cholecystectomy, and all went very well. The patient, her new baby, and the whole family were very satisfied with the care, and there were no postoperative complications. After this experience, my director/educator/leader insisted I write up the case and submit it to the *AORN Journal*, which I did with much trepidation. It became my first published article. She then strongly encouraged me to send a proposal to the Association of periOperative Registered Nurses (AORN) for presentation at the national Congress. This became my first professional presentation. Without this amazing woman's leadership, my own career and perioperative nursing would not be the same today. She went on to become national president of AORN.

The other strong leader that helped me become an effective department chair was my first dean. She had innate knowledge of how to lead, knew the factors that influenced faculty to perform to their best ability, and knew the barriers and boundaries within which nursing schools associated with health science centers must exist today. For example, she taught me realistic methods of handling difficult situations involving students and how

Perioperative Nursing Clinics 4 (2009) ix–x
doi:10.1016/j.cpen.2008.10.011

to work with the independent assertiveness of a professional educator, each of whom was a leader in his or her own right. In my article on educational leadership, it is clear that it has been the main driving force for the modern nursing profession, and educational leaders are still in the forefront of the profession.

An outstanding leader of the nursing profession is Rebecca Patton, the president of the American Nurses Association (ANA) in 2008. Last year, for the first time, she began an affiliation between ANA and AORN, Inc. In reaching out to this large specialty organization, she brought nurses together in an organization affiliation that will allow AORN members to be represented politically and to be eligible for the benefits that ANA provides its members. Through Patton's leadership, AORN and the American Association of Nurse Anesthetists joined ANA at the republican and democrat national conventions during 2008. This joint effort resulted in general increased knowledge and political awareness of needed health care reform.

The need for national leadership and political awareness can be seen in the short article by Oliver. Her clear and concise lists of actions an individual nurse can take to participate in legislative processes are useful. Without an ongoing effort to move the profession forward and assist with improved health care for all people, nursing will fall behind in power and in maintaining an autonomous practice.

Developing clinical leaders is essential to maintain the forward momentum of nursing. The excellent article by Batson (on developing clinical leaders) discusses authentic leadership. All nurses have the capability and opportunity to be a leader. As expressed in the article by Steelman, clinical nurses are leaders, but those in advanced practice roles often have formal administration as their role, lending a greater power and visibility in the leadership role. This person, through advanced education and clinical expertise, has the knowledge to positively influence the quality of patient care, improve staff safety, and implement evidence-based interdisciplinary changes.

Research leaders are making an impact on nursing. You will find concepts and useful information in Cornett and Parson's article, in which they discuss their research on creating a healthy workplace. This promotes an empowerment of nurses that is supported and assisted by middle and higher level managers, which leads to better staff

retention and job satisfaction. Seigel and Kornewicz also wrote about the research viewpoint; specifically about leadership in research and moving nurses from novice to expert in their ability to plan and implement good studies.

Three excellent articles give theories and concepts of leadership. Reineck's unique article demonstrates how leadership can carry from the military to the civilian world and how content and concepts do not change. She gives a framework of five leadership practices. Pacini, who writes on Synergy with leadership development and transformation, also provides a framework. She discusses how the traditional methods of education impede growth and understanding of transformation, which effects outcomes and anticipatory openness to the myriad possibilities available for a leader. Nussbaum wrote the final article on the concepts of leadership. He presents variables not commonly associated with leadership theory. He proposes that each individual's cultural perspective must be considered by a manager to promote the most effective workplace.

As any leader knows, the role cannot be implemented without stress: sometimes considerable stress. Keegan and Barrere discuss strategies for managers to maintain an environment of calmness and support, which is needed by the nursing staff.

Educators, advance nurse practitioners, and researcher leaders contributed to this issue of *Perioperative Nursing Clinics*. As the reader peruses the articles in this issue, it will become clear that there are common elements of leadership, no matter where they are found. Nursing leaders are everywhere, doing everything. They are civilian and military. They are young and old. Some love their jobs, while others tolerate; some are stressed, and some appear oblivious to the pressures and forces they encounter day to day. The reader of this issue will find many things that can help with the professional and personal aspects of life. I hope that you will enjoy this issue as much as I enjoyed putting it together. Happy reading.

Nancy Girard, PhD, RN, FAAN
8910 Buckskin Dr
Boerne, TX 78006-5565, USA

E-mail address
ngirard2@satx.rr.com (N. Girard)

About Face! Five Exemplary Leadership Practices Applied in Contrasting Environments: Military and Academic

Carol A. Reineck, PhD, MSN, MAEd, RN, FAAN, NEA-BC

KEYWORDS

- Leadership • Model • Vision • Challenge
- Enable • Encourage

Question: In the perioperative setting, does leadership have the potential to be as universal as surgical asepsis? This article suggests that the answer is yes. However, suggest to a perioperative nurse that leadership practices in the operating room are no different from those on the battlefield or in a university, and you'll likely get a response such as, "You must not have ever been in my operating room." In other words, perioperative nurses and other clinicians may view leadership as something that differs depending on the setting; or as something only for the corner office. In fact, leadership is an observable attitude that all of us can learn and practice. The effective practice of leadership can help keep patients safe.

This article begins by briefly describing leadership in two markedly contrasting, and familiar environments—the military and academic settings. Five simple, yet exemplary, leadership practices are presented. Brief application of each of the five practices in military and academic settings follows, to illustrate the portability of this framework. The two thrusts of this article are that (1) the five elegantly simple leadership practices are applicable across settings, and (2) they can be learned, practiced, and improved.

It is commonly held that clinical practice poses a challenging context in which to practice leadership. The intensity of patients' clinical presentations, variability in patient arrival patterns, alterations in the pace of work, scrutiny of regulators, and the inherent turbulence, uncertainty, and chaos which characterize these environments may make clinicians wonder if, and how, classic leadership principles and practices can be effectively applied in these extraordinarily complex settings.

Dr. Gerald B. Healy,[1] an otolaryngologist and the 88th President of the American College of Surgeons, stated how the current patient-care environment (described by the Institute of Medicine's reports)[2] requires a team approach. Healy said, "Team training has been proven to be very effective in the airline industry and in the military, and we need to learn from that success."[1] The purpose of this article is to suggest that what is new in leadership is not the content, but rather, the context. That is, while the environment, setting, and circumstances in which teams find themselves may be ever-changing, effective leadership practices remain constant across industries, environments, and settings.

FIVE EXEMPLARY LEADERSHIP PRACTICES

Thousands of leaders and followers were studied in longitudinal and global research on leadership

The University of Texas Health Science Center at San Antonio School of Nursing, 7703 Floyd Curl Drive, Mail Code 7975, San Antonio, TX 78229, USA
E-mail address: reineck@uthscsa.edu

across many continents.[3] Over two decades, investigators analyzed case studies and results from survey questionnaires to uncover five practices common to personal-best leadership experiences. Extensive research findings from administration of the Leadership Practices Inventory revealed that five leadership practices emerged, regardless of the context. Kouzes and Posner's[3] five leadership practices are (1) model the way, (2) inspire a shared vision, (3) challenge the process, (4) enable others to act, and (5) encourage the heart.

LEADERSHIP PRACTICES INVENTORY

"The Leadership Practices Inventory (LPI) was developed through a triangulation of qualitative and quantitative research methods and studies. In-depth interviews and written case studies from personal-best leadership experiences generated the conceptual framework, which consists of the five leadership practices."[4]

Actions that make up these practices were translated into behavioral statements. Following several iterative psychometric processes, the resulting instrument has been administered to over 350,000 managers and nonmanagers across a variety of organizations, disciplines, and demographic backgrounds. Validation studies over a fifteen-year period consistently confirmed the reliability and validity of the LPI and the Five Practices of Exemplary Leaders model. Overall, the LPI has been extensively applied in many organizational settings and is highly regarded in both the academic and practitioner world."[4]

The contrasting environments of military and academic settings offer a sort of operatory in which to see the same five practices at work in vastly different domains. This contrast suggests that this leadership model may be useful in perioperative nursing as well. A brief review of the military and academic environments begins the discussion.

THE MILITARY ENVIRONMENT

Military service members protect and defend the Constitution of the United States from all enemies foreign and domestic. The Army, Navy, Air Force, and Marine Corps operate in an environment requiring integrity, order, and competency. The US Army set forth an acronym, LDRSHIP,[5] to help soldiers remember values most important in tough situations as well as in day-to-day decisions and behaviors. These are:

Loyalty: faithful adherence to a person or unit
Duty: the legal or moral obligation to accomplish all assigned or implied tasks to the fullest of your ability.

Respect: treating others with consideration and honor
Selfless service : putting the welfare of others before your own
Honor: being honest with one's self and truthful and sincere in actions
Integrity: doing what is right, legally and morally
Personal Courage: overcoming fears, danger or adversity while performing your duty

Service members belong to small units (ie, squads and platoons) which are a part of increasingly large units (ie, companies, battalions, brigades, divisions and corps). Generally, effective leadership in the small unit makes it possible for the larger units to successfully accomplish the mission.

THE ACADEMIC ENVIRONMENT

The US Constitution, which our military protects and defends, provides freedom for the pursuit of liberty, such as freedom to learn. The academic environment serves to impart knowledge, develop skill, and increase the ability of students while developing and expanding faculty knowledge. David W. Leslie,[6] Chancellor Professor of Education, The College of William and Mary, declared that "the public wants colleges and universities to be effectively led and accountable for student learning, growth, and development."

The academic environment stands on a traditional and symbolic three-legged stool of teaching, research, and service that requires significant documentation for promotion, tenure, and annual review.[7] Leadership in the academic environment toward the goal of academic quality, involves creating an engaged faculty. While many people traditionally viewed the scholarly work of faculty as primarily teaching and research, more contemporary views[8] have been advanced. Today, scholarship is viewed more richly as: (1) discovery, original research; (2) integration, the synthesizing and reintegration of knowledge; (4) application, professional practice; and (4) teaching, transformation of knowledge.[8] Military and academic environments are markedly different, yet the same five leadership practices are easily applied in both settings. **Table 1** summarizes practices and applications from the military and academia. The point is that fundamental leadership content does not necessarily change when the setting changes.

LEADERSHIP PRACTICE ONE: MODEL THE WAY

The first leadership practice, model the way, involves two commitments—finding your voice by clarifying your personal values, and setting

Table 1
Examples of application of the five leadership practices in military and academic settings

Context		Leadership Practice			
	Model the Way	Inspire a Shared Vision	Challenge the Process	Enable Others to Act	Encourage the Heart
Military	Loyalty, duty, respect, selfless service, 'honesty, integrity, personal courage	Example of Army Communities of Excellence Program	Chain of command; long-term civilian health education and training program	Team training; individual development; officer and non-commissioned officer development programs	Individual and unit awards in a public recognition with tangible ribbons and badges.
Academe	Three pillars: teaching, research, service	Academic centers of excellence	Faculty assemblies, committees and councils	Care for faculty; share leadership with and among faculty	Esteem of building knowledge in self or others. Careful use of public recognition. Focus on the value of the work itself.

the example. Model the way is performed in the military setting with many tangible and intangible indicators. At the most fundamental level, these indicators include wearing the uniform properly, placing insignia correctly, maintaining physical fitness, and rendering proper military courtesy and bearing. At the operational level, modeling the way in the military is characterized by taking care of soldiers: that is, making sure soldiers have the training, equipment, and support to do their jobs effectively and safely; that soldiers have opportunities for promotion and career development; and that soldiers' family members are taken care of Modeling the way in the military is also a matter of exercising unquestioned integrity in every action, because soldiers watch their leaders.

Military service members believe that "People will respect us, gravitate to us, and want to be like us because we are excellent as they define excellence. Said another way, our witness results in great measure from determining the mission essential tasks–the defining and distinguishing tasks in our particular military specialty–and being not only excellent but preeminent at it."[9]

In academe, modeling the way does not bear as many visual indicators as in the military, but some do exist. Granted, there are generally no uniforms except for lab coats and academic regalia at graduation; there are few insignia except medallions worn on special occasions, university patches on lab coats, and pins from honoraries, societies, and schools. One masters-prepared faculty member, nearing voluntary retirement, recently stated that while attending a doctoral graduation, he was moved to plan to apply for doctoral education himself. The point is that sometimes the external indicators like doctoral robes, hoods, and regalia may serve as just the models needed to motivate others.

Model the way in academia involves setting the example in scholarly teaching, research and service; full participation and engagement in the work and governance of the school; sharing leadership; coaching and mentoring others; and demonstrating collegiality with colleagues.

LEADERSHIP PRACTICE TWO: INSPIRE A SHARED VISION

Inspiring a shared vision means envisioning the future and enlisting others in a common vision. Mission and vision are different. In the military, the mission for a unit is an expression of its purpose and is set by requirements of national security. The vision, however, is a preferred future and is developed jointly by the members of the entire unit. One example of inspiring a shared vision is

establishing the Army Communities of Excellenc (ACOE) Program[10] awards. The ACOE Progran recognizes military installations that exemplify ou standing customer service and other importan values. Standards of excellence form the mod to which installations strive. For example, Fo Sill, Oklahoma, won the coveted ACOE award 1994. The hospital on the post, Reynolds Arm Community Hospital, modeled the way for exce lence in military health care for the field artille by providing exceptional health care custom service to soldiers, family members, and retire beneficiaries.

Leaders in academic settings are not necessa ily just the administrators or those in position of a thority, such as deans and directors. For exampl The Center for Creative Change at Antioch Unive sity Seattle celebrated the graduation of its fi cohort of students in June 2005 under an innov tive new design integrating four master's degr programs. Faculty at the Center, leaders ther selves, had a shared vision of an integrated curri ulum to equip students to change the world looking through a systems lens. The faculty reco nized that to realize a new vision, there exist a challenge within themselves and within t team. The following statement summarizes the e perience: "this experience serves as a remind that building a collective vision is not a one-tin endeavor with a definitive endpoint. Rather, a sion is a living imperative, and this makes buildi one an iterative process, with ever-emerging u derstanding and insight that could not have be achieved in the initial inspiration and design."[9]

LEADERSHIP PRACTICE THREE: CHALLENGE THE PROCESS

Challenging the process involves searching opportunities, taking risks, and learning from m takes. An example of challenging the process the military is one from drill and ceremonies. Y have heard the command "About-face!" The p pose of this well-known military command is to mediately change the direction a soldier or grc of soldiers faces. There are two commands– command of preparation and the command of ecution. The command of preparation is "Abou during which command, soldiers prepare to fac the opposite direction. The command of exe tion, "face," directs soldiers to swivel on t toes to achieve the new facing position. It happ within seconds and is orderly and familiar, es cially during drill and ceremonies.

The military is well-known for being able to big things quickly and with precision. Challeng the process in the military is done through chain of command. When an opportunity for improvement presents itself, soldiers gather information needed to brief superiors and offer clear-cut alternatives, each with advantages and disadvantages outlined.

Another example of challenging the process is the investment the military makes in graduate education, such as the Long-Term Civilian Health Education and Training Program. Officers apply, are board-selected to attend, and return to the military with new ideas to improve processes.

In academia, challenging the process is not so orderly. Academic freedom brings with it the empowerment to bring the most current knowledge into the classroom and to employ chosen teaching strategies, subject to the review of other faculty. Faculty members challenge the process through innovations in teaching, conducting research to solve problems, and by engaging with other faculty around curriculum revision. Faculty senates, councils, and assemblies are other forums where the process is challenged at the governance level.

LEADERSHIP PRACTICE FOUR: ENABLE OTHERS TO ACT

Enabling others to act includes two commitments: fostering collaboration and strengthening others. Lieutenant General (retired) Bruce Fister[11] reflected that, "While commissioned officers decide, direct, and establish the command climate, sergeants "make it happen." Enabling others to act in the military is primarily a function of officers' clear direction and getting out of the way to let the noncommissioned officers and soldiers get the job done in ways that work best.

In academe, enabling others to act is a matter of supporting the faculty, who in turn, teach and support students and engage in their scholarly work. John Millet[12] stated "The key element in the academic process and in the academic community is the faculty. There is no other justification for the existence of a college or university except to enable the faculty to carry on its instructional and research activities. Without a faculty higher education has no reason for being." Enabling others to act in academe is a matter of creating the environment in which faculty can thrive. Thriving faculty are innovative in their teaching, focused on the future, engaged in scholarship, serve the community, and are collegial with each other.

The 2008 Association of Perioperative Registered Nurses President Susan K. Banschbach[13] cited the importance of mentoring emerging leaders, "With each generation, rebirth is critical because clinging to the past diminishes the future." This is an excellent example of enabling others to act through mentoring.

LEADERSHIP PRACTICE FIVE: ENCOURAGE THE HEART

Perioperative nurses work exceptionally hard. They rightfully become exhausted. Encouraging the heart includes acts of caring that range from dramatic gestures to simple actions. Two commitments in encouraging the heart are recognizing contributions and celebrating the values and victories by creating a sense of community.

The military is especially devoted to this practice. Service members receive individual awards and badges for performance of duty. Unit awards are also given, to recognize superior performance of entire groups of soldiers.

Unlike military leaders who submit award recommendations very frequently, have formal ceremonies to present the awards, and who offer tangible ribbons and badges signifying the awards, academic recognition is handled with somewhat more reserve and restraint. Generally, it is the work itself that brings reward in academia. Publishing an article; authoring a book; receiving a grant, fellowship, or appointment; being promoted in academic rank; receiving the grant of tenure, or receiving the esteem of colleagues or students are examples of rewards. It is generally the case that faculty members' work is more likely to be recognized than the faculty member themselves. Teaching, research, and service are the missions of academia. Advancing understanding of phenomena is the reward.

SUMMARY

Five classic leadership practices[3] seem to be universally effective. The leadership practices are: (1) model the way, (2) inspire a shared vision, (3) challenge the process, (4) enable others to act, and (5) encourage the heart. These five practices form a classic, straightforward, and tested set of best-practice leader behaviors noted and appreciated by followers world-wide. Examples of the leadership practices applied in two markedly contrasting settings–the military and academia–offer the insight that the content of leadership does not change; rather, the context or setting is what changes.

The perioperative nursing workforce demonstrates the five leadership practices in their care for millions of patients each day. The National Center for Health Statistics reported that 44.9 million inpatient surgical procedures (including interventional cardiology, endoscopic, and radiographic diagnostic procedures) were performed in 2007.[14] To accomplish the clinical care, leadership is critical. Leadership helps integrate the efforts of the entire surgical team amid simultaneous pressures to achieve the expectations of the access, quality, and cost triad. The five leadership practices provide a simple and useful framework to guide perioperative nursing leadership.

REFERENCES

1. Healy GB. Presidential address: competence, safety, quality: The path of the 21st century. Bull Am Coll Surg 2007;92(12):9–13.
2. National Academy of Science. Institute of Medicine. To err is human: building a safer healthcare system. 1999.
3. Kouzes JM, Posner BZ. The leadership challenge. 3rd edition. San Francisco (CA): Jossey-Bass; 2007.
4. Sashkin M, Rosenbach W. A new vision of leadership. In: Taylor R. editor. Contemporary issues of leadership, 1998 contemporary issues of leadership. Boulder (CO): Westview Press; 1988. p. 79. Available at: http://media.wiley.com/assets/463/74/lc_jb_appendix.pdf. Accessed November 14, 2008.
5. Corps of discovery: United States Army. The seven army values. 2003. Available at: http://www.history. army.mil/LC/The%20Mission/the_seven_army_values htm. Accessed June 30, 2008.
6. Leslie D. (in Wergin, J.) Leadership in place: how academic professionals can find their leadership voice. Bolton (MA): Anker Publishing; 2007. p. xvi.
7. Diamond R. Preparing for annual review. Bolton (MA): Anker Publishing; 2004.
8. Boyer E. Scholarship reconsidered: priorities of the professoriate. Princeton (NJ): The Carnegie Foundation for the advancement of teaching; 1990.
9. Hower M, Hormann S. Creative redesign for change. Chapter 5. In: Wergin J, editor. Leadership in place. Bolton (MA): Anker Publishing Company, Inc.; 2007. p. 76–106.
10. Headquarters, Department of the Army (DA). DA Pamphlet 600–45, Army Community of Excellence (ACOE) guidelines Washington, DC. 1991.
11. Fister B. Letter from the Executive Director. Connected. Englewood (CO): Officers' Christian Fellowship; 2008. p. 2.
12. Millet J. The academic community: an essay of organization. New York: McGraw-Hill; 1962.
13. Steiert MJ, Banschbach SK. President's message. Passing the baton. AORN J 2008;87(4):711–3.
14. United States National Center for Health Statistics Centers for Disease Control. Available at: http://www cdc.gov/nchs/fastats/insurg.htm. Accessed April 1, 2008.

Developing Leaders Through the Healthy Workplace Intervention

Patricia A. Cornett, EdD, MS, RN[a],*,
Mickey L. Parsons, PhD, MHA, RN, FAAN[b]

KEYWORDS

- Healthy workplace • Healthy workplace intervention
- Participatory action research • Future search conference
- Empowerment • Engagement • Participatory leadership
- Leader development

The role of the nurse manager is one of the most important and challenging in health care. They are responsible for management of the day-to-day business of the nursing unit and expected to serve multiple constituents; including patients, families, physicians, and executives. They are also depended on to lead their staffs in provision of safe and culturally sensitive patient care—all in the face of a pandemic nursing shortage and aging registered nurse (RN) workforce.

The scope of competencies required to fulfill such expectations is enormous. Jennings and colleagues[1] conducted a comprehensive literature review of competencies. The analysis differentiated nursing leadership and management competencies and, as a result, Jennings and colleagues stated that the vast array of competencies identified verified assertions that leaders and managers are expected to be all things to all people.

They identified 10 categories for leadership competency and ranked them according to the number of times the competency was identified in the literature reviewed: personal qualities, interpersonal skills, thinking skills, setting the vision, communicating, initiating change, developing people, health care knowledge, management skills, and business skills. Ten categories for management competency were also identified and ranked in the same manner: interpersonal skills, personal qualities, thinking skills, management skills such as planning, organizing, communicating, business skills, health care knowledge, human resources management, initiating change, and information management. Personal qualities, interpersonal skills, thinking skills, and communicating were the most frequently cited competencies in both the leadership and management categories. Setting the vision in the leadership category and management skills in the management category rounded out the top five competencies. In the final tally, the intersection of leadership and management competencies was 96%. Ambiguity persists. Harvard Business School professor David Thomas points out during an interview by Blagg and Young, that "increasingly, the people who are the most effective are those who essentially are both managers and leaders."[2]

Kondrat's[3] study of operating room (OR) managers' competencies support that notion. He identified two competency sets that distinguish superior OR managers from competent ones. Competencies in the human and leadership categories were more indicative of a superior OR nurse manager, along with managing fiscal and material resources.

Mackoff and Triolo[4] studied 30 outstanding long-time nurse managers in six settings. They

[a] Solucion International—Workforce and Workplace Solutions, 133 Watts Lane, Canyon Lake, TX 78133, USA
[b] The University of Texas Health Science Center at San Antonio School of Nursing, San Antonio, TX 78229-3900, USA
* Corresponding author.
E-mail address: solucioninternational@gmail.com (P.A. Cornett).

identified 10 signature behaviors of these outstanding managers. Five of the behaviors contribute to Jennings and colleague' most frequently identified leadership competency of "personal qualities." They are (1) generosity, finds gratification and joy in others' development; (2) ardor, conveys excitement about staff, colleagues, and leaders; (3) boundary clarity, cultivates strong internal boundaries and models such; (4) reflection, leverages lessons from experience; and (5) self-regulation, suspends judgment before acting.

The second most frequent competency Jennings and colleagues identified was "interpersonal skill." This is a good fit for two of Mackoff's behaviors: attunement, shows regard for the individual and the appreciation of each person's contribution; and affirmative framework, generates positive expectations. Thus, 7 of the 10 behaviors identified by Mackoff correspond to the top two competencies found by Jennings and colleagues.

It is noteworthy in Jennings and colleagues findings that two important areas of both leadership and management work were largely ignored. Developing a healthy work environment was mentioned only six times as a leadership competency and only two times as a management competency. According to Jennings, this reflects a poor fit between identified competencies and the current need to improve work environments. Healthy work environments have been aptly described by the American Association of Critical Care Nurses,[5] the American Hospital Association,[6] the Institute of Medicine,[7] and The Joint Commission.[8] The other important area of competence for leaders is dealing with people's differences by letting conflicts surface. Conflict resolution was identified as important for superior OR nurse managers in Kondrats' study. In Jennings' study, collaboration was addressed more often than conflict.

Given the scope of expectations, it is not surprising there is a paucity of frontline nurse leaders able to manage the equivalent of a small business, attend to all constituents needs, and create healthy workplace environments that are enriching to staff and subsequently all constituents.

PARTICIPATORY LEADERSHIP

Why is a healthy workplace so important? Healthy workplaces are characterized as empowering environments where shared leadership and participatory management exist among all staff.[9] The relationship of workplace empowerment with better recruitment, retention, job satisfaction, and employee engagement,[10–12] and with higher organizational commitment,[13,14] has been established. Personal empowerment characterized by

autonomy, confidence, and feeling one can mak a difference in the organization has also bee demonstrated.[15]

Kanter's theory of structural empowerment de scribes the formal lines of power in an organizatio as (1) access to information, (2) access to re sources to do the job, (3) opportunities to lea and grow, and (4) support.[16–19] Alliances with su periors, peers, and subordinates are the co structs of informal power. The mandate for upp management according to Kanter is to ensure sta has access to those formal lines of power. In tur staff who believe those lines are open for them fe empowered. Additionally, empowerment is infl enced by the informal power of alliances with su periors, peers, and subordinates.

Review the leadership or management sectio in bookstores and one will find a multitude books describing the alphabet soup of leadersh qualities: benevolent, emotional intelligenc transformational, visionary, quiet, participator servant, effective, and trusted. There is a pletho of information on what leaders do and how su cessful ones have done it. The messages are co sistent and clear. No matter what the endeavo a leader's success—meaning the organizatio success—is about the leader engaging the hea and minds of employees by allowing them to cr ate their own story; their own future.[20] An empo ered and trusted staff is an engaged staff and th drive productivity up and cost down.[21]

HEALTHY WORKPLACE INITIATIVE

Helping leaders engage the hearts and minds their staffs so that together they create their o story and future is the essence of a nursing u based, capacity-building process titled Healthy Workplace Intervention that promo shared leadership, participatory change and e powerment.[22] The building of this desired fut is accomplished using participatory action search, a social research model that is perform by a team comprised of a professional action searcher and members of an organization seek to improve their situation.[23] In the Healthy Wo place Intervention, the team is the nursing staff, the nurse manager, interdisciplinary st and two professional action researchers.

Future search conferencing (FSC), a plann conference method whereby people can bri differences in status, position power, work exp ence, gender, and hierarchy by working as pe to achieve shared goals and fast action enab the team to (1) systematically explore proble and issues, (2) formulate powerful and soph cated accounts of the situations, and (3) de plans to manage such.[22,24] It is also experiential learning for the nurse manager in creating participatory and shared leadership.

Transitioning to shared leadership for a nurse manager whose personal experience has primarily been a hierarchical model requires a willingness to learn to lead from the middle: learning to create and maintain the structure for staff access to the formal lines of power and to strengthen their informal power of alliances with the manager, their peer group, and subordinates. Leading from the middle is throwing open the doors of power and depending on the collective brilliance of the group to envision, define, refine, implement, evaluate, and celebrate what needs to be done. It is not just leading from the front, giving orders and directives. Nor is it just leading from the back, pushing one's staff toward predefined goals. Shared leadership is the re-engineering of the nurse manager role, learning to be a leader of leaders.

METHODOLOGY

The methodology used to implement participatory action research is FSC methodology. Nineteen acute care units in seven different tertiary care hospitals in a metropolitan area participated in a six-phase Healthy Workplace Intervention.

In phase one, an introductory meeting was held by the nurse executive, nurse manager, and action researcher to describe the intervention and plan staff meetings to present the opportunity to create their future.

In phase two, a one and a half day FSC was conducted off campus in a retreat-like setting. Staff in each patient care unit were invited to attend the FSC for their unit only. Size of FSC groups ranged from 12 to over 50 participants depending on the size of the unit, number of staff, and type of service offered such as medical nursing unit or a perioperative department. The steps in this FSC process were: establish objectives for the conference and establish ground rules for working together, and develop a shared history and a shared desired future vision. Then a Mind Map, the gestalt of the unit's desired future was created to give form to the unit's vision. Priorities were then ascertained and participants voted on the top three priorities and developed detailed action plans for each, resulting in the start of actualizing their vision.

In phase three, a six month booster conference was held with staff, managers, and researchers to determine what had been accomplished thus far, what had not been accomplished and why, and how to finally get there.

Phase four was the twelve-month follow-up conference where action teams presented their outcomes, reflected on lessons learned, and establish the priorities and action teams for the next year.

Phase five was the annual unit meeting to select new priorities and develop plans for the ensuing year. At this point, the nurse manager assumed the role of facilitating the annual meeting. The final phase was sharing outcomes and best practices through the formal hospital-shared governance councils and boards. For a full description of the theoretic framework and intervention see Parsons.[22]

LEADER DEVELOPMENT

Tulgan states the primary management myth today is the myth of empowerment which holds that the way to empower professionals is to leave them alone to do their work.[25] With the broad scope of leader-manager competencies to accomplish, nurse managers need guidance and support. The best leaders are those who learn proven techniques, practice them until they become skills, and continue to practice until they become habits.[25]

Development of the leader begins in phase two, during the planning meeting with the nurse executive, nurse manager, and action researcher. Even at this early stage, leadership styles of nurse managers are evident. For example, nurse managers with a personal transactional leadership style accept the Healthy Workplace Intervention as just another project to take on and accomplish. Some telling comments are, "Let's pick the dates for the FSC and I'll select the staff I know will be willing to participate" or, "How do I keep the naysayers away? They'll put a negative spin on everything." At this point, the manager may actually identify staff by name and give examples such as, "She'll go right to her favorite surgeon and tell him she's being pulled out of his room for two days to go attend some planning meeting." This becomes a teachable moment where the nurse executive or action researcher can explain that exclusion actually enhances any informal power-base of such negative-attitude staff members. Then, using an action learning[26] approach, the researcher may ask questions of the manager to elicit information about results the manager has experienced with the current methods of managing staff members with primarily negative attitudes. Continuing with a series of questions, the researcher guides the manager to uncover her or his underlying assumptions and link them to the actual outcomes.

Phase one is an opportunity for the action researcher to assure the nurse manager he or she is not alone in this change initiative. The Healthy Workplace Intervention process depends on the involvement of as many staff members as possible because people are less competitive and more collaborative when they are working on the joint goals that are their story, their future.

The second phase, the FSC, is a concentrated exercise in communication, aiding the nurse manager in moving to a more shared, delegation-style leadership. During the conference, the action researcher's role is to facilitate the process and role-model interpersonal competency behaviors for the nurse manager such as fostering free discussion, actively listening, clarifying major and minor points, assisting the group's adherence to their self-established behavioral ground rules, modeling the communication competency behaviors of allowing conflict to surface, acknowledging emotionally-laden issues, and posing questions to individuals and the group as a whole.

During the initial steps of the FSC, the researchers coach the nurse manager by encouraging her or him to articulate to the group (interpersonal competency) the challenges and expectations he or she perceives from all constituents (setting the vision and health care knowledge competencies) and to express her belief in their collective brilliance to design solutions (developing people competency). Those solutions that are beyond the unit's scope of control may still be within their scope of influence and the nurse manager can assist them in forwarding their recommendations to the organization's executives (setting the vision competency).

During the later action-planning steps, participants self-select into specific action planning teams for the top three priorities. During several two hour segments, each group does the detail planning work of identifying the what, how, by whom, by when, and evaluation of outcomes. The nurse manager is not a member of any team but is advised to float among the planning groups to observe, support, and give input (thinking skills, initiating change, and business skills competencies). Managers with a tendency toward command and control behaviors in an environment that calls for shared leadership can be coached in the moment. Guidance is given on relationship-development behaviors (personal qualities, interpersonal skills, and communication competencies) that engender trust such as openness, giving information in a way people will perceive the manager does care about them and their ideas, and whose intent is a win-win scenario for everyone. The desirable outcome is a spirit of transparency that results in staff feeling their manager is real, genuine, and cares about them.[21]

The action teams report out to the larger group following each intensive workgroup session in order to receive feedback and gain consensus that they are moving in the intended direction. These interactions are high value in building trust among peers and subordinates because people are given time to get to know each other's motives, values, knowledge, and skills.

In some cases, a team may have veered from the original intent. When that occurs, questions to clarify why the group moved in such a different direction are most useful. Encouraging the nurse manager to respond in such a manner or role modeling this behavior by the action researchers demonstrates the meaning of leading from the middle. Lunch and dinner breaks are ideal times for the action researchers to meet with the nurse manager for reflective thinking and discussion which are essential for her or him to operate creatively to form a new understanding of connections between what is done and its consequences.[27]

During the subsequent action team meetings that occur during the six-month period between the FSC and the six-month booster conference the manager continues to practice the behavior with his or her staff individually and with the action teams. Skills become habits and a steady growth in leadership competence is the ultimate outcome. By the one-year conference, the nurse manager has truly moved to a higher level of competency particularly in the top five leadership competencies identified by Jennings: personal qualities, interpersonal skills, thinking skills, communicating and setting the vision, and making development of a healthy work environment a reality.

SUMMARY

Thompson[28] states that the goal of shared leadership is to create an environment of interdependence that values the expertise of staff at all levels. Shared leadership is not a competency; is a re-engineered leadership role that requires superior competence in communication and trust building. The Healthy Workplace Intervention a hands-on, experiential-learning opportunity participatory leadership for nurse managers with consistent support and guidance from the action researchers. It is also a means for staff to begin the journey to become leaders in their own right and to create their own future. The outcome is an empowered staff that lead change and create their own future in an environment of high trust, supported by a manager who has captured the hearts and minds—a Healthy Workplace.

REFERENCES

1. Jennings B, Scalzi C, Rodgers J, et al. Differentiating nursing leadership and management competencies Nurs Outlook 2007;55:169–75.

2. Blagg D, Young S. What makes a good leader? Harvard Business School, Working Knowledge. April 2; 2001.

3. Kondrat B. Operating room nurse managers – competence and beyond. AORN J 2001;73(6):1116–30.

4. Mackoff B, Triolo PK. Why do nurse managers stay? Building a model of engagement. Part 1. J Nurs Adm 38(3):11–124.

5. American Association of Critical Care Nurses (AACN). AACN Standards for Establishing and Sustaining Healthy Work Environments. A Journey to Excellence. Am J Crit Care 2005;14(3):187–97.

6. American Hospital Association (AHA) Commission on Workforce for Hospitals and Health Systems. In our hands. How hospital leaders can build a thriving workforce. Chicago: American Hospital Association; 2002.

7. Institute of Medicine. Keeping patients safe. Transforming the work environment of nurses. Washington, DC: National Academies Press; 2004.

8. Joint Commission on Accreditation of Healthcare Organizations. Health care at the crossroads: strategies for addressing the evolving nursing crisis. Oakbrook, IL: JCAHO; 2001.

9. Parsons M, Clark P, Marshall M, et al. Team behavioral norms: a shared vision for a healthy patient care workplace. Crit Care Nurs Q 2007;30(3):213–8.

10. Lashinger J, Havens D. Staff nurse empowerment and perceived control over nursing practice. J Nurs Adm 1996;26(9):27–35.

11. Moore S, Hurchison S. Developing leaders at every level. Accountability and empowerment actualized through shared governance. J Nurs Adm 2007; 37(12):564–8.

12. Lashinger H, Finegan J, Shamian J, et al. A longitudinal analysis of the impact of workplace empowerment on work satisfaction. J Econ Behav Organ 2001;4:527–44.

13. McDermott K, Laschinger J, Shamian J. Work empowerment and organizational commitment. Nurs Manag 1996;27(5):44–8.

14. Lashinger J, Finegan J, Shamian J. Promoting nurses' health: effect of empowerment on job strain and work satisfaction. Nurs Econ 2001;19(2):42–52.

15. Spreitzer G. Social structural characteristics of psychological empowerment. Acad Manage J 1995; 39(2):483–504.

16. Lashinger H, Wong C, Greco P. The impact of staff nurse empowerment on person-job fit and work engagement/burnout. Nurs Adm Q 2006;30(4): 358–67.

17. Lashinger H, Finegan J. Empowering nurses for work engagement and health in hospital settings. J Nurs Adm 2005;35(10):439–49.

18. Kanter RM. Men and women of the corporation. NY: Basic Books; 1977.

19. Kanter RM. Men and women of the corporation. NY: Basic Books; 1993.

20. Tichy N. The leadership engine. NY: HarperCollins; 2002.

21. Covey SMR. The speed of trust. NY: Free Press; 2006.

22. Parsons M. Capacity building for magnetism at multiple levels. A healthy workplace intervention, part 1. Top Emerg Med 2004;24(4):287–95.

23. Greenwood D, Levin M. Introduction to action research. Social research for social change. Thousand Oaks (CA): Sage; 1998.

24. Emery M, Purser R. The Search conference: a powerful method for planning organizational change and community action. San Francisco, (CA): Jossey-Bass; 1996.

25. Tulgan B. It's okay to be the boss – be a great one! J Nurs Manag 2007;38(9):18–24.

26. Origins of action learning. Available at: http://www.IFAL.org.uk. Accessed June 24, 2008.

27. Dewey J. How we think: a restatement of the relation of reflective thinking to the educative process. Boston: D.C. Heath; 1933. [Original work published 1909].

28. Thompson P. Patient safety: the four domains of nursing leadership. Nurs Econ 2005;23(6).

Perioperative Nursing and Politics: Where Do You Start?

Joanne D. Oliver, RN, BSN, CNOR

KEYWORDS

• Perioperative • Nursing • Legislation • Politics • Negotiate

When I began my career in perioperative nursing, I never dreamed I would be testifying before a Senate hearing committee or communicating with my legislators on a regular basis. I was just helping out a colleague who had the political "bug." I learned that to ensure the direction of our profession, we had to learn to inform, educate, negotiate, and stimulate others to do the same. This article discusses specifics on each of these items as they relate to perioperative nursing and legislation.

INFORM

When we inform, we must start by informing ourselves about the issues and how they relate to perioperative nursing as well as nursing in general. This process also means asking the question "How will this affect us as a potential patient?" One can start by performing the following:

- Read legislative advocacy updates.
- Know the current legislative priorities of the Association of periOperative Registered Nurses (AORN).
- Join AORN grassroots.
- Research various Web sites or "Google" specific terms that may need clarified.
- Check with your state nursing association.
- Offer to assist in development of an alliance of various other professional nursing organizations.
- Read journals.
- Stay up to date on AORN's position statements.
- Investigate the Web sites of other allied health organizations to keep abreast of new issues.

- Stay informed on who your congressional representatives are.
- Offer yourself as a resource on perioperative nursing issues to your local, state, and national congressional members.
- Talk to their staff and find out potential health issues they might be concerned about.
- Take time out to attend your state lobby day when your legislature is in session.
- Drop by your congressman's office in Washington, DC.

Performing just a few of these steps in the beginning will help stimulate you to get started. Remember also that staying informed is a lifelong process just like your practice, and that experience in nursing is a never-ending process.

EDUCATE

While you are constantly informing yourself, you will begin to share this information with others. In this way people will become informed, excitement will be generated, and issues that may have been overwhelming before will start to become resolved. Who do you educate and what do you as an individual do? Remember that an election can be influenced from the actions of one or the actions of many. The following are some suggestions:

- Hold a political in-service for your staff.
- Write a paper for a journal.
- Ask a political leader in your city to come and speak at your AORN meeting.

28 Champions Colony, West Houston, TX 77069, USA
E-mail address: jolivertx@comcast.net

Perioperative Nursing Clinics 4 (2009) 13–15
doi:10.1016/j.cpen.2008.10.007

- Offer to bring a politician to your operating room suite for a visit.
- Speak at a school (nursing, high school, junior high, elementary, or senior citizen's home).
- Participate in a trade fair.
- Conduct an open house to promote perioperative nursing.
- Participate in state council activities.
- Look up pending bills.
- Learn how to read and interpret a legislative bill.
- Look up references in a bill to another bill. (Do not just assume these were okay.)
- Request a proclamation from your individual city hall.
- Attend the city hall meeting. (They must read the proclamation, and you may be on local television.)
- Present your side of an issue to your legislative representative or aide. (Be sure to leave them a copy of your presentation or at least a list of the key points you want them to remember.)

NEGOTIATE

It is easy to discover an issue that is of concern to you. Currently, one of our primary priorities is making sure we have a registered nurse for every patient undergoing surgery. Our local AORN chapter used this slogan to post on a freeway billboard during perioperative nurse week! When you negotiate, you want to think about what items are absolutely not negotiable versus what parts of the proposal you might be able to live with. In negotiation, there is always some give and take. Your aim is to ensure you do not give up what you cannot live with. It is hoped that you end by creating an atmosphere where everyone wins. You negotiate every day in your normal life. You just have to learn how to do this in the legislative arena as well. The following are some tips to remember:

- Assemble all of the stakeholders for the negotiation meeting. Do not waste time negotiating without them. Although you may come to what you think is a great agreement, a key stakeholder who has not had any input might block any progress you have made.
- Prepare an agenda to discuss, with an expected outcome, and stick to it.
- Send all participants a list of the agenda and attendees expected.
- Set a timeframe to address specific areas.
- Look at your biggest concerns first. (If you cannot agree on some of the basic principles, the details would be a waste of time.)

- Bring appropriate documentation or references to support your viewpoint.
- Be prepared to give examples or provide stories to support you position.
- Set up the next steps to complete for any negotiation settled.
- Follow-up with a summary of discussions and agreements by providing documentation that will itemize the end results.
- If legislation is to be written or congressional representatives need to respond, be sure to keep them informed of the results of your stakeholders meeting.
- If lobbyists are involved, they can be your biggest support to further negotiate and educate other legislators.
- If a response is not received in an appropriate period of time, follow-up.
- Do not publish your strategies while you are still in the negotiation process.

STIMULATE

Everyone has different things that motivate them into action. The biggest issue often suggested as a deterrent to participating is a lack of time or interest. How can you stimulate someone to get involved? This task has been an age old process to try to figure out. I like to think of this aspect as "one minute management." Most folks will bend over backward for you with some praise and will aide in participation. Sending out a general "we need volunteers" message is okay but does not often stimulate someone to participate. A personal call to an individual telling them you really need them and supporting them when they do get involved gets a lot more results. The following tips may be helpful:

- Appoint a team for your legislative committee. (Creating relationships with your elected officials as well as their aides take time. Be sure to retain some of your seasoned nurses and continue to add new nurses as well.)
- Invite your participants to an orientation meeting as part of another fun function.
- Hold a meeting at your home or schedule a conference call. (The Web site accessed at www.freeconferencecall.com is an inexpensive way to establish a conference call number.)
- Stage an audience participation activity at a practice trial or hearing.
- Create a team leader concept with a seasoned nurse and new nurse.
- Take that new nurse with you to a meeting with legislators.

- Schedule a trip to a lobby day, city council meeting, political action committee, or local Republican or Democratic committee.
- Participate in the promotion of a candidate for office.
- Go listen to a state hearing committee meeting on any health care issue.
- Plan time to share information gained.
- Provide practice sessions for presentations.
- Coordinate with your nursing and hospital association to address issues of concern for both.
- Listen to your nursing colleagues to see what they need or how suggested legislation would affect their practice.

Involving nurses in active legislation is a rewarding opportunity that all of us must be involved in. There is power among nurses that can mold the future direction of health care. We must learn to inform ourselves, educate others, negotiate for the betterment of our patients, and stimulate our colleagues to get involved. We are facing a drastic shortage in nurses across the country and in perioperative nursing in particular. Our elected officials are faced with thousands of issues, and they cannot be experts on every subject. It is up to us to offer our experience and give simple examples that will bring our points to the forefront. We need to protect our practice, develop our resources, expand our opportunities, and remember that any one of us might be the next patient affected under any new legislation. If you want the very best for you and your family, take it upon yourself to get involved and share your knowledge and experience with others. Listen, learn, and share. Your time and efforts will be well worth the benefits received.

Leadership: Unrecognized Variables to Success

George F. Nussbaum, PhD, RN, CNOR

KEYWORDS

- Diversity • Counseling • Concept of time
- Group dynamics • Organizational culture

Cultural beliefs and norms develop through a lifetime of the conditioning and experiences of each individual. Common understandings about body language cues, the concept of time, the expression of intense feelings, and the hierarchy of relationships in the workplace are foundational in each specific culture. Individuals within cultural groups become, to a greater or lesser degree, acculturated through their formative years. They continue to reinforce these constructs through association with similar members and through their own experiences.[1–3]

These patterns persist in the work environment, and as such create leadership challenges in communication based upon differences in fundamental cultural norms.[4] Workplace behavior-norm expectations are those behaviors established in institutional tradition and values for the good order and conduct of all members.[4] Collectively, these codes of conduct regulations are intended to create a new culture and normative behavior for all employee members. The degree of change required to meet and adapt to the expectations of these norms may vary considerably among individual members.

There may be an assumption that fundamental and universal group norms exist in the work environment, and that these are central themes for all participating members. This concludes that the members comprise a homogeneous group and that norms are accepted as a given. Select group behavioral norms belonging to group members may be of greater significance than others and may be considered more central than perceived by members from differing groups.

There are cultural differences between members of differing races, specifically between Blacks and Whites. "Diversity in its broadest sense applies not merely to a collection of people who are alike in some ways and differing in others, but also to intangibles—ideas, procedures, and ways of looking at things."[5]

Much has been written in nursing literature regarding the care of culturally different patients. There are, however, few studies that consider culturally acquired norms as a potential influence on communication in the workplace.[6,7] Other studies consider cultural aspects of patients that are cared for in the medical environment, but no study has considered the cultural influences on communication between the medical personnel.[6] Specifically, there are no research-based studies that explore diversity and behavior-norm issues in the professional nursing and paraprofessional workforce. Unintended communication barriers and miscues may result from behavioral norm expectation differences. If substantial differences regarding these issues exist, then knowing, understanding, and appreciating these differences may create a more harmonious and more efficient work environment.

SYMBOLIC INTERACTIONISM

Symbolic interactionism is a theoretic framework that helps to illustrate the complexities of leadership communication challenges. This theory focuses on the nature of social interaction.

The views expressed are those of the author and do not represent the views of the U.S. Army, Department of Defense, or Uniformed Services University of the Health Sciences.
Uniformed Services University of the Health Sciences, 4301 Jones Bridge Road, Bethesda, MD 20814, USA
E-mail address: george.nussbaum@tma.osd.mil

Perioperative Nursing Clinics 4 (2009) 17–22
doi:10.1016/j.cpen.2008.10.009

There are three basic assumptions of symbolic interactionism:

Members of society, individually and collectively, respond on the basis of meanings that things represent to them. That is, individuals as a product of a unique cultural background attach meaning to communication cues and act on the basis of that meaning. For each member, the world is interpreted through the use of symbols, such as language, gestures, and nonverbal stimuli in the process of interaction. Members act on their understanding and interpretation of meaning that is derived from symbolic interaction.

The process of interacting aids in establishing a common meaning. Meaning for an individual emanates through the actions and interactions with other individuals. The symbolic interactionist perspective is that individuals are able to act because of their agreement on the meanings attached to the communication symbols and cues in their environment.

The process of understanding meaning is both assigned and modified through interpretation that can change, be redefined, and realigned.[8] There remains the assumption that individuals have a freedom of choice, yet that choice is constrained by societal and cultural norms. Within this context, individuals have the capacity to synthesize the symbolic use of oral communication and gestures to create and communicate meaning and a common response in the interaction with others. The interpretation of stimuli provides new meanings and new responses that serve to actively shape the interpretation of meaning.[8]

Symbolic interactionism contributes a theoretic perspective to describe how individuals from differing cultural backgrounds interpret meaning during the communication process with others, and how the process of interpretation leads to behavioral responses in specific communication episodes. Assumptions underlying symbolic interactionism have excellent utility in the design of qualitative studies.[9]

CULTURAL PERCEPTIONS OF TIME

The construct of time is perhaps one of the most significant diversity-related phenomenon that is least appreciated when considering cultural issues in the workplace. The orientations toward time vary greatly across cultural groups. The aspect of time is widely reported in the literature as being varied among peoples, yet it is not discussed in leadership-team building or diversity-training content as critically problematic.

Time, as a unique cultural norm, is a primary element in how peoples are united or isolated from one another. Time, when treated as a variable to be understood in the study of cultural norms serves to identify how activities in life are organized, how priorities are established, and how experiences are categorized. The cultural understanding of time provides the mechanism to determine the efficiency or lack thereof with respect to competence, effort, and achievement. Cultural norm rules governing time provide an intangible measuring mechanism for determining respect issues, trust values, how people feel toward one another, and a significant determinate for whether or not they can get along.[10]

Time-Orientation Perspectives

There are three time-orientation perspectives, as follows:

Linear-separable: this orientation views time as including the past, present, and an infinite future, with specific emphasis on future. Time is considered separable in that there are quantifiable, specific units with defined beginnings and endings for categorical events.

Circular time-orientation: in this orientation cultures experience time as determined by repeated cycles of activities, such as rotating seasons, agricultural activities, and birth, life, and death.

Procedural: in this orientation, time becomes essentially irrelevant allowing that behavior is activity-driven and will take the amount of time it takes to complete.[11]

The perioperative work setting, often comprised of multiple ethnic subculture members, clearly favors a linear orientation to time. Evidence of this is noted with the extreme emphasis on scheduled start times for workplace activities, a preoccupation with deadlines, due dates, promptness, and mission accomplishments through short- and long-range planning. This orientation is typical in the normal life activities for white Americans but not so, in general for African Americans, Hispanic-Americans, and Asian-Americans, whose time orientations tend to be circular, procedural, or a combination of both.[11–14]

Illustrating this in the African American culture, the frequent absence of a specific end time for social or religious events. The meaning of this cultural-specific norm is that scheduled start times for events and appointments are treated by many with a great deal of flexibility.[11,14] Many workplace individuals from the African American culture have an orientation toward circular and procedural time. It may be more important for individuals from traditional African American culture to be "in time;" that is, in synchronization with the perceived natural rhythm of life rather than to be "on time," which is imposed time for many events, including work.[12]

Most white Americans have a propensity for a "monochromic" time orientation, meaning a more rigid "one thing at a time" planning and activity schedule.[14] Monochromic time orientation includes a strong affinity for rigid clock watching and an on-time approach to all of life's events. Tradition-oriented black Americans are "polychromic" with respect to time orientation.[14] Polychromic time orientation is defined as being involved in many activities simultaneously without regard to clock time. In this orientation, the activities and the relationships at hand take precedence over defined schedules. The potential for cultural-norm conflict and diversity tension clearly exists when tradition-oriented polychromic members are subjected to the rigidity of a monochromic work environment.[13–15]

CULTURAL ALLOWANCES OF EXPRESSIVENESS

Communication norm expectations vary greatly between White and Black cultures. White male-dominated organizations expect that discussions will remain calm and generally unemotional. Voice inflection is expected to be low and well modulated, with the maintenance of a polite atmosphere. Intense, emotionally charged and argumentative challenges are rare or nonexistent by expectation. Violations of this communication code are usually dealt with by formal or informal disciplinary action, especially if the individual expressing the anger, hostility, or perceived violent emotion is in a subordinate role.[12]

In the White culture, individuals are expected to restrain or suppress their emotions. From childhood, white Americans are taught that if you don't have anything nice to say, don't say anything at all. Therefore white Americans, especially in the workplace, conform to the behavioral norm of suppressing anger feelings and conform to the acceptable code of restraining expressiveness.[12]

A common description of American communication and leadership assumes a workforce as a homogeneous culture. This workgroup is described as:

Problem oriented: Each event in the workplace is viewed as a problem to be solved. There exists an assumption that problems need solutions and that is the basis of work and reality.

Direct: Supervisors and workers are expected to value the time of the other and consequently skip the small talk. Expressions such as "Get to the point," "Get down to business," "What is the point?" or "What's the bottom line on this?" are common statements in the predominately White business environment.

Explicit: What is stated in words is what is meant. Skill is required to learn how to state your point. The context of the message is located in the verbal statement, while the nonverbal signals, such as gestures and facial expressions, take on a lesser value in the perception of meaning. American business culture places little emphasis on context of the conversation and high trust in the words used in the message.

Personal: Commonly, Americans' relationships do not run deep. Superficial topics, such as where one lives or has lived, sports likes and dislikes, and other actions and experiences are explored to find a basis for relationships.

Informal: Americans tend to dispense with explicit formality in conversations and move quickly to an informal contest. This is best illustrated by the use of first names early in a relationship. This degree of informality is uncommon in other cultures.[16]

A very different viewpoint illustrates that the American culture is not a homogenous mixture with identical norms for all members. The behavioral norm for a White employee would be to keep silent on contentious issues, or to at least refrain from argument. The behavioral norm for African Americans would generally be the opposite; namely, if individuals have a position on an issue, they are obliged to speak up. The interpretation from the Black members' view is that silence signifies agreement. The Black cultural norm is supportive in the expression of strong feelings and values the abilities of individuals to regulate their own emotions. White cultural norm requires that impulses toward self-assertion be restrained. In those events, when anger boils over and is expressed strongly, the White individual has a sense of having lost control. White American individuals practice throughout life the subtle art of aggressive/expressive self restraint.[17]

Black Americans, to be perceived in the White work arena as socially acceptable, often suppress their cultural norm of expressing their true feelings. This constraining behavior is known as "fronting."

Whites are seldom aware of the fronting behaviors because restraint of these emotions is part of the White cultural norm. Blacks must make a day-to-day effort to match the unnatural lingua franca effort to contain their emotions "in what they regard as a racially hostile environment."[15,17] Lack of passion on issues is regarded by Blacks as insincerity. This is especially difficult as the Black culture fully grants the liberty to express emotions.

Other cultural studies reveal that degrees of expressiveness among Blacks is frequently condemned and misunderstood by White teachers and police. These cultural misunderstandings often lead to unwarranted and undeserved punishment, when a true cultural understanding of Black expressive norms would have been more helpful.[15]

OCULESIC AND KINESETIC (PARALINGUISTIC) VARIANCES

Leadership communication is a complex phenomenon that is seldom mastered or understood, even in the closest of working relationships. The range of opportunities for communication miscues begins with word selections to convey a message through voice volume, tone, kinesecis, and oculesics. Kinesics, or body language, refers to gestures and important body movements that are incorporated into a speech act to convey messages. There are five major categories of kinesic behavior:

Emblems: nonverbal acts that have direct verbal translations, such as those found in greetings and gestures of agreement.
Illustrators: movements tied to speech, which serve to illustrate the spoken word.
Affective: displays, such as facial signs, indicating happiness, surprise, or fear.
Regulators: acts that maintain and regulate the act of speaking, indicating when a speaker wants to start talking or to relinquish the floor to another.
Adapters: signs originally linked to body needs, such as wiping your brow or lip biting.[18]

Oculesics, or eye behavior, is a source of intense communication potential, as well as a source for damaging communication miscues between individuals within and between cultural groups.[19] Eye contact between culturally different members varies widely. Black and white Americans have near opposite eye contact patterns. "African Americans generally have greater eye contact when they are speaking than when they are listening. Whites reverse the pattern, showing greater eye contact when they are listening than when

they are speaking."[12] This creates a situation whereby Whites and Blacks are staring at one another when the Black member is speaking. Whites are inclined to "interpret direct and sustained eye contact... as a sign of intensity and passion."[12]

Traditional African Americans typically avoid eye contact as a sign of showing respect, especially anyone in an authority position. This is frequently perceived by Whites as a sign of inattention, lying, or disinterest.[20] "To most white Americans, eye contact indicates attentiveness, respect, and confidence.... If the listener looks away, however, may be interpreted as disrespect, disinterest, a lack of confidence, or dishonesty."[14]

In the workplace setting, when eye contact that is otherwise correct within the culture of the individual is misperceived during interaction, feelings of mistrust, misjudgments of attentiveness, and disrespect evolve from the communication. These tragic communication miscues serve to deepen and enforce incorrect stereotypical ideas between Black and White workforce members, and further complicates the ability of leaders to lead an effective organization.[3,12–14]

Eye behavior serves six communication functions:

To influence attitude change;
To indicate a degree of attentiveness, interest or arousal;
To display emotions;
To guide interaction;
To establish boundaries on power and status;
To create impressions in others.[19]

PERFORMANCE COUNSELING

Supervisors dread counseling employees for poor performance or behavior issues. This counseling often results in negative relationships between employees and supervisors and represents a significant leadership deficit. Conflicts with and among employees represent one of the least recognized and the largest reducible costs in organizations.[21] Workplace conflicts from any source, including leadership's lack of understanding of cultural differences and communication errors, are expensive both in money and wasted time.

Supervisors often fail to counsel employees on performance issues because they fear potential consequences. These consequences include:

Fear the employee will become angry or react violently.
Fear the employee will resign. In many instances, the question becomes whether it would be better to have a marginal employee or none at all.

Fear the counseling will be ineffective.

Concern the employee will cause chaos among other team members.

Worry among supervisors that the employee will not respect their authority.

Concern the employee will seemingly agree with the counseling, yet sabotage the organization in other ways (eg, taking frequent sick days, failing to document legitimate patient charges used during procedures)

Fear the employee will illuminate the supervisor's leadership failures.

Concern the employee will point out inconsistencies and the unfairness of selectively counseling them, while others are not reprimanded.[22]

Relationships between staff members and departmental leaders are vitally important within organizations. Conflict can add stress to an already complex environment. The lack of consistent counseling skills in organizations represent productive time wasted worrying, gathering facts, writing counseling statements, conducting counseling, and managing the aftermath. This lack of skills results in supervisors making bad decisions, agreeing to compromises that ultimately exacerbate the problem. Supervisors who repeatedly make bad decisions and demonstrate a lack of leadership ability lose the trust and respect of staff members. Employees will seek less stressful environments with solid leadership.[22]

COUNSELING DIFFICULTIES

The act of counseling an employee for poor performance or unsuitable behavior can be unpleasant for everyone involved. By avoiding the task, department members suffer the consequences in a variety of ways. Forgiveness in organizations is not customary policy. Performance or behavior issues normally result in formal counseling events. These events place an employee in a no-win situation. As a result of a negative counseling document, employees believe there is little hope for future promotions or salary increases. Counseling sessions are rarely productive and often are frustrating for all parties involved unless forgiveness is possible.[22]

There is an incorrect perception on the part of leaders; they often make the statement they "have a problem employee." This implies that the problem belongs to the leader and that correcting the difficulty is the leader's responsibility. Employees often react to counseling with denial, anger, threats, tears, and other means to minimize

the damage. In the absence of understanding, mercy, or forgiveness, the employee has little to lose. As long as the employee can make the leader the one who has the problem, the employee can partially survive in the job. At the very least, the employee can hope to minimize the situation. The perceived task of the leader is to gather sufficient pertinent facts, document them well, and confront the problem employee. The problem employee will either correct the behavior, resign, or choose not to correct the behavior and be fired. In any case, the supervisor no longer will have the problem. The fact is, the supervisor never had the problem — only perceived it as such. It is the employee that has the problem, as well as the responsibility to correct the problem. The leader's task is to bring the issue to the surface and allow the employee the opportunity to resolve it.[22]

Effective counseling requires an exchange of opinions with the intent to reach a decision and form a deliberate plan to resolve problems. When forgiveness and restoration of harmony is possible, the negative consequences of this type of counseling can be avoided. Leaders must allow employees to admit their mistakes, to discuss and commit to making the required changes. In exchange, the leader must work with the employee to maintain a positive relationship. True forgiveness implies that when the issue is completely resolved, all associated counseling documentation is destroyed.[22]

The concept of forgiveness is counterintuitive in American organizational culture; however, when the true ownership of a problem is recognized and the responsibility placed accordingly, excellent results are possible. Reaching a deliberate, nonpunitive, nonthreatening plan of action rarely happens in the absence of a mechanism that allows the employee to adjust course with dignity, respect, and future opportunities.[22]

GROUP-THINK

As paradoxical as it may sound, leaders must learn how to manage agreement more frequently than they manage conflict situations. "...the inability to cope with (manage) agreement, rather than the inability to cope with (manage) conflict, is the single most pressing issue of modern organizations."[23] "Organizations frequently take actions in contradiction to what they really want to do and therefore defeat the very purpose they are trying to achieve."[24] When workers fear they will be ostracized or punished if they appear to present opposition within the group, they will simply go along just to keep the peace. Leaders must consciously create a workplace where people are encouraged to voice their true opinions and encouraged to disagree when they believe individuals in organizations provide false, public support to plans they know are impractical or dysfunctional, adding to group decisions that are meaningless and often costly to organizations.

Leaders must be fully aware of catastrophic group-think dynamics to prevent false agreement in the group environment. It is crucial that leaders strive to create a work environment where group members are not fearful of speaking out and disagreeing with issues that may negatively impact true organizational cohesiveness and financial effectiveness.

Leadership is an increasingly complex process in workplaces with employees with differing cultural family heritages. Leaders are expected to be subject matter experts in the disciplines they are to lead. Values that may include trust, duty, competence, loyalty, integrity, and respect are among the required characteristics for an ideal leader. However, leadership is more than the sum of the leader's values and attributes. Leaders must learn to ask the right questions about the employees they are to lead. The knowledge of followers' cultural norms with respect to their concepts of time, allowable expressiveness, and paralinguistic nuances are significant in avoiding unintended communication miscues and the resulting problems that develop. Being prepared with skilled counseling techniques and the ability to understand the complexities of group dynamics will aid leaders in achieving personal and organizational success.

REFERENCES

1. Bar-Tal D. Group belief: a conception for analyzing group structure, processes, and behavior. New York: Springer-Verlag; 1990.
2. Lustig MW, Koestger J. Intercultural competence: interpersonal communication across cultures. (2nd edition). New York: Harper Collins College Publishers; 1996.
3. Ting-Tommey S. Communicating across cultures. New York: Guilford Publications, Inc.; 1999.
4. Moskos CC, Butler JS. All that we can be: black leadership and racial integration the army way. New York: HarperCollins College Publishers, Inc.; 1996.
5. Thomas RR. Redefining diversity. New York: American Management Association; 1996.
6. Giger JN, Davidhizar RE. Transcultural nursing: assessment and intervention. (2nd edition). St. Louis (MO): Mosby-Year Book, Inc.; 1995.
7. Purnell L. Workforce cultural diversity. Surg Serv Manag 1996;2:26–30.
8. Blumer H. Symbolic interactionism perspective and method. Englewood Cliffs (NJ): Prentice-Hall, Inc. 1969.
9. Benzies KM, Allen MN. Symbolic interactionism as a theoretical perspective for multiple method research. J Adv Nurs 2001;33(4):541–7.
10. Hall ET. The silent language. New York: Bantam Doubleday Dell Publishing Group; 1981.
11. Cox T Jr. Cultural diversity in organizations: theory, research and practice. San Francisco: Berrett Koechler Publishers; 1994.
12. Fine MG. Building successful multicultural organizations: challenges and opportunities. Westport (CT): Quorum Books; 1995.
13. Henderson G. Cultural diversity in the workplace: issues and strategies. Westport (CT): Praeger; 1994.
14. Henderson G. Our souls to keep: black/white relations America. Yarmouth (ME): Intercultural Press, Inc.; 1999.
15. Shipler DK. A country of strangers: blacks and white in America. New York: Random House, Inc.; 1997.
16. Stewart EC, Bennett MJ. American cultural patterns a cultural perspective. [revised edition]. Yarmouth (ME): Intercultural Press, Inc; 1991.
17. Kochman T. Black and white styles in conflict. Chicago University of Chicago Press; 1981.
18. Ekman P, Friesen W. The repertoire of non-verbal behavior: categories, origins, usage, and coding. In Malmkjaer K, editor. The linguistics encyclopedia (2nd edition). New York: Routledge; 1969. p. 283.
19. O'Hair D, Friedrich GW, Wiemann JM, et al. Competent communication. (2nd edition). New York: St. Martin's Press, Inc.; 1997.
20. Gudykunst WB, Kim YY. Communicating with strangers: an approach to intercultural communication. (3rd edition). New York: McGraw-Hill Companies, Inc.; 1997.
21. Dana D. Managing differences: how to build better relationships at work and home. Prairie Village (KS): MTI Pub; 1999;13: p. 15–21.
22. Nussbaum GF. Counseling: establishing a culture forgiveness. AORN J 2007;86(3):415–22.
23. Harvey JB. The abilene paradox: the management of agreements. New York: Organizational Dynamics American Management Association. 1988. p.17–4.
24. Harvey JB. The abilene paradox and other meditations on management. Lexington (MA): Lexington Books; 1988. p. 18.

Developing Clinical Research Projects: Novice to Expert

Jeanne H. Siegel, PhD, FNP*, Denise M. Korniewicz, PhD, RN, FAAN

KEYWORDS

- Clinical research • Evidence-based practice
- Novice to expert

Nurses today are faced with multiple tasks and institutional demands that require continued change in the clinical environment. Because of concerns raised by national and international studies associated with the cost of health care, patient safety factors, and new regulations associated with reimbursement, nurses at the bedside are being asked to improve patient care outcomes. Therefore, most staff nurses lack the skills associated with evidence-based approaches or data-driven results. In fact, most clinicians must be reeducated about their role within the organization and as an active member in gathering data, participating in clinical research forums, or working with multidisciplinary teams to promote new clinical treatments.

Clinical research is a necessary part of clinical practice to assure improvements in patient care. In an ideal world, research and clinical practice occur together, with research being the mechanism that results in improved clinical practice, thus providing a springboard to identify clinical research problems.[1] Nurse clinicians are in a unique position to identify the nursing problems that become the core of nursing research studies. In addition, nursing (American Nurses Association), regulatory (Joint Commission on Accreditation of Hospitals), and government (Agency for Health Care Administration, National Institutes for Health) organizations continue to promote evidence-based practice (EBP) guidelines and participate in transdisciplinary projects promoting clinical research. Transdisciplinary research is defined as a full investigational partnership, credit sharing, and recognition of a disciplines' unique contribution to the area under study.[2] To be competent and full partners in translational research, nurses as clinical experts must develop the necessary research skills.

The data collected during research enable clinicians to monitor the success or failure of treatment or prevention interventions in a logical and systematic manner. Nurses can be involved in clinical research through using qualitative and quantitative methods to objectively evaluate acute or chronic interventions performed at the bedside. However, to conduct meaningful and reliable research, a step-by-step process that will lead to significant results must be understood. This article provides knowledge of the developmental stages (novel to expert) needed to conduct clinical research projects in an acute care environment.

NOVICE TO EXPERT: DEFINING THE CLINICAL RESEARCH MODEL

One method to promote change and encompass clinical research within the clinical environment is to use Pat Benner's "Novice to Expert" model.[3,4] Embedded in the model are various roles (**Table 1**) that can assist clinical researchers with developing research at the clinical unit level. Principles associated with clinical research for the novice may include becoming involved with a journey of discovery. *Discovery* in the clinical setting may include an understanding of how to use evidence-based guidelines from a simple review of literature or participation in research-use teams. Often novice learners may become the most valuable member of the research team because they are eager to learn new skills. However, use of a research mentor

University of Miami, School of Nursing and Health Studies, P.O. Box 248153, Coral Gables, FL 33124, USA
* Corresponding author.
E-mail address: jsiegel@miami.edu (J.H. Siegel).

Perioperative Nursing Clinics 4 (2009) 23–29
doi:10.1016/j.cpen.2008.10.006

Table 1
Definitions of novice to expert, examples of clinical research

Description	Definition[3]	Clinical Research Examples
Novice	Little experience; requires rules and broad guidelines to organize	Recruits participants for the study. This beginner researcher has valuable clinical knowledge and assessment skills to target appropriate individuals to participate in a specific study. With direction, the novice can collect data. Clinically, novice performs protocol interventions and treatments.
Advanced beginner	Focuses on the immediate present; relies on protocols, and forecasting is limited by experience	Experienced in data collection and the area of research being conducted. Identifies potential participants and with direction begins to consent participants for the research study. Participates in the development of research instruments, surveys, and data collection tools. Clinically, performs protocol interventions and treatments. Serves as a resource for novice researchers for protocol concerns.
Competent	In same or similar job for 1 to 2 years; views actions in terms of long-range goals or plans of which consciously aware	Meets with potential participants to obtain informed consent. Understands the need to protect participant's right to be informed and to make informed decisions about participating in a research study. Responsible for protecting the confidential information provided by research participants. Assists in identifying the financial needs of a research study including equipment and personnel.
Proficient	Perceive situations as whole rather than separate parts; see the global picture	Serves as project director overseeing the day-to-day direction on the study. Directs and monitors the students, research assistants, and other research staff responsible for collecting or entering data. Participates in the statistical analysis of data and the publication of findings. Participates in obtaining funding for research projects through grant writing and contact with potential research sponsors.
Expert	Respond to the particular situation; focus on salient issues; operate from a deep understanding of the total situation	Serves as principal investigator (PI) with overall responsibility for the research study, including Institutional Review Board decisions and oversight responsibilities. When necessary the PI decides when to remove participants from a study or to end a study. Oversees the publication and presentation of research findings in peer reviewed journals and research symposia. Manages grant funding in collaboration with the organization's budget manager (accountant). Serves as the researcher in residence at a hospital or health care facility. Mentors research work throughout the health care facility. Serves as PI if necessary to develop inexperienced researchers. Mentoring new and inexperienced researchers at all levels. Attracting new clinical researchers by demonstrating the benefits (to the profession and the clients) of research findings.

to foster their clinical inquiry must be part of the infrastructure.

The second level of learner in Benner's model includes the advanced beginner. In clinical research, this may be a nurse who has been involved in working with others on a clinical research project or a nurse researcher. Examples of advanced beginners include nurses who have instituted clinical protocols and have been involved in understanding the differences in patient outcomes associated with defined clinical protocols. Other examples include development of a simple survey to be used with other nurses or health care worker staff to determine best practices.

The third level of learner includes the competent clinician. This staff member has been working 2 years or more, has embraced the goals or initiatives of the unit, and continues to provide leadership to junior staff. Examples of the competent clinician in research include knowledge about the research process, data collection methods, and conducting clinical studies with other researchers. The competent clinician is an important team member because they can be trusted to teach more junior staff and be mentored into a clinical research project director.

The fourth level of learner is the proficient staff member. The important attribute associated with this learner is the ability to view the whole picture. For example, the proficient staff member has an understanding of the research projects; is fully engaged in designing the project, collecting data for the project; and is engaged in writing protocols associated with the project. The proficient clinical staff members are essential members on the unit because they lead other members toward understanding the research process and promote changes based on clinical findings.

The final learner is known as the expert clinical researcher. This person is fully engaged in research, such as a doctorally prepared clinical nurse researcher. Competencies of the expert include a terminal degree in research (PhD), and knowledge about how to develop a research project. This individual also understands how to obtain grant funding, conducts research, and is fully engaged in multiple research studies. Often clinical staff nurses are not at this level; rather, the institution has made a commitment to research and has used doctorally prepared clinical researchers to assist staff members who can conduct research projects at the unit level.

NOVICE TO EXPERT: APPLYING THE MODEL

Nurses involved in clinical nursing research help to further develop the discipline and profession of nursing. Nurses who are involved at any level (novice to expert) of research help to develop and use EBP and best practice guidelines[1] that provide credibility and accountability in the nursing profession. Furthermore, through using data derived from EBP projects, nurses can establish cost-effective best practice interventions.[5] Clinical nurses can provide research ideas within the domain of nursing and test interventions (derived from research) at the bedside. Whether a nurse is at the novice or expert level of knowledge about research methods, successful clinical research requires new or enhanced skills to develop a clinical research problem, design a research study, collect data, and interpret the results.[1,6]

As a clinical research leader, working with clinical staff nurses during each of these phases is important. One way to enhance these nurses' knowledge and skill is to provide discussion groups about the research process through having them identify the similarities and differences of the research process with the nursing process. Nurses are excellent at identifying the nursing problem and, as the facilitator of research, the clinical research leader's role is to provide the environment of inquiry and coach the staff during each phase.

OVERVIEW OF THE RESEARCH PROCESS

All research studies involve a five-phase process, including the conceptual phase; the design and planning phase; the empiric phase; the analytic phase; and the dissemination phase.[1] Each phase has unique challenges that must be overcome by the research team.

Identification of the Research Problem

The conceptual phase draws heavily on the knowledge of the researcher to identify and formulate a clinical problem. During this conceptual phase, the researchers identify a problem, determine the research purpose, and determine what questions the research will be designed to answer. This phase consists of conceptualizing or formulating the research question through completing a review of the literature for background information and determining the body of literature associated with the proposed idea.[1,6] A complete review of current literature, commonly the past 5 years, is necessary to identify trends and identify gaps in the knowledge. Often, nurses ask original research questions that are rooted from clinical experience, such as questions about nursing care, cost, best-practice or evidence-based guidelines, product evaluation, adverse events, or patient care outcomes. A review of literature (ROL) provides data about what is already known about the area of interest. Access to a library containing medical and nursing references and journals is crucial for all nurses involved in the research process. A good ROL will also show the gaps in knowledge. Furthermore, an extensive ROL will allow researchers to familiarize themselves with the current knowledge base and nursing practice. Nurse researchers in essence become experts on the current state of knowledge for the nursing problem under study.

A clinical research project begins when a clinical research problem and research questions are envisioned by a clinical practitioner or researcher. Defining and redefining the clinical question is important because it becomes the driving force of the clinical research project. Furthermore, it helps develop the type of research design needed to create the research protocol or the blueprint of a research project (**Box 1**).

Designing Clinical Research Projects

The research design and planning phase encompasses developing a research team, selecting a research design, developing study procedures, determining the sampling frame, and creating a data collection plan.[1] This phase consists of researches making decisions on the methods they will use to address the research questions designed in the conceptual phase. Members of the research team are identified and their responsibilities clearly defined during the design and planning phase. The most important phase of a research project is the planning phase. The more complete and thought out the planning, the less likely unforeseen problems will arise and the more successful the project will be.

The members of the research team should consist of the principal investigator (person who developed the project), unit clinical staff, data

collectors, data entry personnel, and statistical personnel. A research team may have nurses at various levels of research expertise. Each nurse learns from those with more experience to improve their skill in the research process.

A research design will differ between quantitative and qualitative research methods. In a quantitative proposal, the methods should describe the consent procedure, setting, sample, data collection tools and process, and data analysis plan. The quantitative research design must focus on controlling components that will determine how accurate and interpretable the collected data will be. A researcher must decide the type of study (interventional versus comparison), how the data will be collected (detailed data collection plan), methods to control other clinical issues, research sites, units, and data analysis (statistical methods). Additionally, the sample size is important to determine so that all results can be accurately analyzed.

In qualitative research, after informed consent is obtained, a process of questions and observations will prompt responses from the research participants that are analyzed later using methods such as content analysis, axial coding, or description. In a qualitative design, decisions about how to best collect the data, from whom to collect it, when to collect it and when its collection ends evolve over the course of the study.[6] This emergent design allows decisions to be made on an ongoing basis based on what has already been learned.

In the quantitative and qualitative research methods, the researcher attempts to enhance the study validity. The *study validity* is the ability of a researcher to make accurate conclusions from the data that were collected and analyzed. *Validity* refers to the degree to which a study accurately assesses the concept that the researcher is attempting to measure.[7] In quantitative research, validity is evaluated by looking at the interval validity, external validity, construct validity, and statistical conclusion validity.[1]

Human Subjects Review

Clinical research is closely supervised and monitored because of ethical concerns about research on human subjects. All studies, with the rare exception of some performed to improve quality of patient care within the quality assurance departments of medical establishments, must undergo Institutional Review Board (IRB) scrutiny and approval.[1] IRBs were developed as a result of the 1978 National Commission for the Protection of Human Subjects of Biomedical and Behavioral Research. The goals of the commission were

---

Box 1
Example of research problem, purpose, and research questions

Problem: Increasing rates of childhood obesity in the United States.

Purpose: To identify factors associated with development of obesity in junior high school students.

Questions: What factors show a statistically significant association with obesity in children in this population? Is the rate of obesity different in males versus female junior high school students?

identify basic ethical principles that should guide conduct in research studies and to develop guidelines based on the principles identified.[5] The commission report, the Belmont Report, served as a model for the development of guidelines for ethical research. The three primary ethical principles on which standards of ethical conduct are based include beneficence, respect for human dignity, and justice.[6]

Most investigators can locate an IRB at their hospital or institution. The IRB will evaluate the research protocol for recruitment, protection, and informed consent of research participants. Some studies that include the development and administration of medications also require approval from the U.S. Food and Drug Administration (FDA) before a clinical research study can begin. In addition, all researchers must complete a Human Participants Protections course and be knowledgeable of the Health Insurance Portability and Accountability Act (HIPPA). Research in the clinical area must comply with the confidentiality requirements of HIPPA, including procuring HIPPA release of information from the participants, unless waived by the IRB.

Analyzing Clinical Research Data

During the analysis phase of research the investigator identifies the relationships between the variables in the research study, eventually answering the research question asked during the beginning of the research project. In quantitative research, statistical methods are used to determine the results of the study after all data collection has ended. Data collected in quantitative research studies consists of numerical values that measure certain patient outcomes. Examples include nominal (gender, blood type, marital status), ordinal (ordered according to some criteria), interval (specific rank order with equal distance between them), and ratio (scales have a rational meaningful zero). Depending on the research question and the final outcomes of the study, the type of data collected for the study depends on the initial research question.

Descriptive statistics assist the researcher in organizing the data into tables to determine the frequencies or percentages associated with the results.[6] Sophisticated computer software packages are available to calculate various statistical tests once data is entered into a database. For new researchers, it is wise to collaborate with a statistician or another researcher well versed in statistical methods to serve as a mentor through this process.

In some methods of qualitative research, data collection and analysis may occur simultaneously, with the collection of data shedding light on new avenues of exploration. Data collection may continue until all avenues are exhausted and no new information is obtained. When data collection yields no new data, investigators use fixed methods to compare responses in verbatim transcripts of interviews or field notes looking for patterns and relationships that will answer the original qualitative research question.

Communicating and Using Research Findings

How do researchers communicate findings to other health care professionals? Dissemination of the findings and conclusions of any research project, including those with negative and nonsignificant findings, should be disseminated to other health care providers and researchers. Nursing research is of little use if only the investigators and research team are aware of the findings. Therefore, all investigators have a responsibility to publish and present research findings to disseminate the research findings and propose new questions for future research. Several avenues exist to publicize research findings, including publication in peer-reviewed journals, poster presentations, and symposia or conferences. Involvement with clinical organizations or honor societies are a good entry point for presentations, posters, and funding opportunities.

Implementing Clinical Research Projects

The characteristics of honesty, the ability to motivate others, a positive outlook, good communication skills, an approachable demeanor, knowledge, and support were all ranked as having high importance in being a successful nurse researcher. The nurse's goal should be to change practice through research by implementing interventions that have shown beneficial outcomes in research. The following sections provide an overview of how to implement a successful research project.

Obtain a coat of armor

Research is rewarding, but not easy. A great deal of work must be done before nurses can collect the first bit of data. A researcher must be determined to overcome any obstacles. In addition, nurses may use various excuses to resist participating in research. As a new researcher, these barriers may appear insurmountable. Persistence and tenacity will overcome initial resistance to any well-planned research project. For example, if the clinical site the nurse planned to use is unwilling or unable to host the research project, an alternate clinical site may be necessary. Because most nursing departments are trying to embark on the "Magnet Journey," suitable research sites should not be an issue.

Prepare to take off: take your first steps

Nurses should develop a committed research team by using clinicians who will help see the research project become a reality, and obtain buy-in from the nursing administration and supervisors early in the project's development. The resources should be found in the nurse's department and facility. Is a nursing researcher in residence? Does the local university have a School of Nursing?

Creating a relationship with available researchers to serve as mentors can be beneficial to both parties. Is a training program or seminars available at the school?

Nurses should ask other researchers for advice on sites, budget, computer and software, statistical support, and funding. Research requires funding to develop the project, purchase materials, and cover participant costs. Does the organization have funding available? Is someone present who assists researchers in writing and obtaining research funding?

Include the nursing staff at the research site during the initial planning process. The support and acceptance of a research project by the staff is crucial to the success of a project. When developing a budget, breakfast or lunch breaks should be included to discuss the project with unit staff and emphasize how their role or participation will make it a success. The staff should have frequent (daily) contact from the research team. Recognize staff for their contributions to the project and watch for future researchers that can be mentored.

Begin the journey: learn from others as you grow

Nurses should develop a written proposal for their research projects. Include the members of the research team in the process. The proposal should include an introduction to the problem, including the purpose of the study; a short summary of the review of literature that supports the need for this research (background and significance); and the methods to be used to complete the project, including research questions, sample characteristics, data collection, and analysis. The proposal should be reviewed by another researcher who is knowledgeable of the type of study planned. Nurses should keep an open mind; research projects are group projects. Using the best ideas from all members of the research team and

outside consultants will result in a better proje[ct] than using the ideas of just one researcher. Add[i]tionally, nurses should be prepared to take cri[ti]cism. Often others will have a different idea [or] suggest other ways to develop the project. Nurse[s] should not be afraid to listen and rewrite to im[im]prove the proposal.

Enjoy the rewards: become the expert

The most significant reward should be the recog[ni]tion that you have contributed to the body [of] knowledge of your profession. The professio[n] does not grow or advance without continued co[n]tribution to the academic capital (knowledge). T[he] clinical researcher also feels a sense of accom[im]plishment and growth by observing staff nurse[s] who have mastered new skills that were n[ot] a part of their basic education. Often several [of] these individuals decide to further their educati[on] and return for a higher degree. Most institutio[ns] will fund trips to present or further the develo[p]ment of research programs for their nursi[ng] departments. This ability to travel and collabora[te] with researchers around the world can be satisf[y]ing and enlightening.

Nursing researchers, over time, strive to b[e]come experts in their research field. Researche[rs] should look for opportunities to enhance th[eir] knowledge and skills in their area of interest, a[nd] should frequently review the literature for curre[nt] developments in their area of research. Th[ey] should present their research findings and lea[rn] from others at research presentations and beco[me] active in the professional organization that rep[re]sents their area of practice.

SUMMARY

Clinical practitioners at all levels of nursing ha[ve] a responsibility to their clients to deliver the b[est] EBP. Despite the many challenges of nursing [re]search, the rewards are great for the research[er] and the clients they serve. The expectations fr[om] government and nursing organizations are cl[ear] in their desire to see nursing research within th[eir] own practice, and participation in translatio[n] multidisciplinary research.

The future agenda of nursing research is [at] the bedside," because the goals of the next m[il]lennium demand bringing the science to [the] bedside. Nurses are essential participants [to] shape the future of nursing by actively par[tici]pating in the clinical research that promo[tes] the quality of care. It is time that resista[nce] stops and research becomes embraced in [the] daily workload of the nurse.

REFERENCES

1. Whittemore R, Melkus GD. Designing a research study. Diabetes Educ 2008;34(2):201–16.
2. Grey M, Connolly CA. Coming together, keeping together, working together, interdisciplinary to trans-disciplinary research and nursing. Nurs Outlook 2008;56:102–7.
3. Benner P. From novice to expert: excellence and power in clinical nursing practice. Upper Saddle River (NJ): Prentice Hall Health; 2001.
4. Burns N, Grove SK. Understanding nursing research. 3rd edition. Philadelphia: Saunders; 2003.
5. Nieswiadomy RM. Foundations of nursing research. 5th edition. Upper Saddle River (NJ): Pearson Prentice Hall; 2008.
6. Ploit DF, Beck CT. Nursing research: principles and methods. 7th edition. Philadelphia: Lippincott, Williams & Wilkins; 2004.
7. Burns N, Grove SK. The practice of nursing research: conduct, critique, and utilization. St. Louis (MO): Elsevier; 2005.

Holistic Serenity: Transcending the Stresses of Leadership

Lynn Keegan, PhD, RN, AHN-BC, FAAN[a], Cynthia Barrere, PhD, RN, AHN-BC[b],*

KEYWORDS

• Holistic • Serenity • Leadership • Stress

Nurse leaders have a critical role in shaping nursing and health care. In all areas of nursing, the visions of nurse leaders and their ability to implement those visions improve health care. The support of dedicated and energetic nurse leaders is an essential aspect in the creation of health care environments to foster caring and healing. Whether the nurse is a new leader transitioning to a first-line management role, a clinical nurse specialist assuming a clinical leader role, or an established leader in an executive role, it is important for him or her to practice effective stress management strategies to maintain an atmosphere of calmness and to provide the inspiration needed to guide and support nursing staff, especially in the midst of tension-filled and challenging situations.

Stress is rampant in many environments in our society, especially in the workplace. It can have a major impact on the lives of individuals and negatively affect their well-being.[1] Stress is directly related to illnesses such as heart disease, anxiety disorders, high blood pressure, coronary artery disease, cancer, respiratory disease, accidental injuries, cirrhosis of the liver, immune system alteration, and suicide.[2–6] These illnesses are the leading causes of death in the United States. In addition to causing illness, stress worsens other conditions such as multiple sclerosis, diabetes, herpes, mental illness, alcoholism, drug abuse, and family discord and violence.

Stress not only affects personal well-being but also is responsible for a portion of the financial costs of the health outcomes of stress in medical expenses and insurance. The medical costs alone have been estimated in the United States to be well over 1 billion dollars per year. Stress costs industry approximately 150 billion dollars per year in increased health insurance outlays, burnout, absenteeism, reduced productivity, costly mistakes, poor morale, high employee turnover, as well as family, alcohol, and drug-related problems.

Stress is not always negative. When managed correctly, harmful stress-related outcomes can be minimized or prevented. Stress is a normal aspect of life that all individuals experience at some level. At times, the stress response can be helpful, for example, by increasing one's alertness during a complex critical care delivery or during a general management meeting in which selected nurse leaders present a quality improvement idea for consideration by the entire management team. The problem occurs when stress that exceeds a productive level interferes with one's ability to think, remember, and focus on tasks. Stress that is ineffectively managed and that remains too high for too long can contribute to physical and psychologic illnesses. This article presents an overview of stress followed by thoughts for nurse leaders on selected ways to deal with stress

Dr. Keegan is one of the founders of the holistic health focus in nursing. She has authored or coauthored 18 books and numerous scholarly journal publications. Work by Dr. Barrere includes holistic research, publications, and presentations focused on palliative end-of-life care/education, spirituality, the care of stroke patients, nurse-patient communication, and the integration of holism into BSN nursing curricula.

[a] 315 Shade Tree Lane, Port Angeles, WA 98362-9292, USA
[b] Department of Nursing, Undergraduate Nursing Program, Quinnipiac University, 275 Mount Carmel Avenue, Hamden, CT 06518, USA
* Corresponding author.
E-mail address: cynthia.barrere@quinnipiac.edu (C. Barrere).

Perioperative Nursing Clinics 4 (2009) 31–41
doi:10.1016/j.cpen.2008.10.008

from a holistic perspective through self-evaluation and transcendence.

WHAT IS STRESS AND HOW DOES IT OCCUR?

Stress is a state of tension created when an individual responds to pressures from work, family, or other external sources, as well as those internally generated from self-imposed demands, obligations, and self-criticism. In many cases stress can become a cumulative and chronic disorder if the individual does not learn to change the behavior to decrease the rising stress level. Stress accumulates over time until a state of crisis is reached and symptoms appear.[7] These symptoms may manifest themselves in the body as well as in the mind. Early symptoms of stress can be seen as irritability, anxiety, impaired concentration, mental confusion, poor judgment, frustration, and anger. As stress accumulates, individuals often develop physical symptoms. The most common physical symptoms include muscle tension, headaches, low back pain, insomnia, and high blood pressure.

Stress is our response we when are in a situation that evokes the sympathetic system, that is, the flight or fight response.[8] When the body receives a stimulus from a stressor, that stimulus is reported to the hypothalamus. The hypothalamus then gives an order to adjust the body according to the stimulus. The autonomic nervous system becomes active and selected hormones increase. Because the autonomic nervous system and hormones are activated, there is some stimulus on the circulatory system, the respiratory organs, the digestive organs, the urinary organs, and bones, muscles, and skin. There is also an effect on the metabolism of internal secretion and nerves. In nature, this type of response helps animals release adrenalin and flee or attack a predator or prey; however, in the work setting, the release of hormones and chemicals does not serve as well the potential purpose for which it was once useful. Most individuals pay a psychologic and physical price when their internal balance is disrupted by a perceived threat, change, or transition. Several physiologic changes occur, including increases in muscle tension, heart rate, and blood pressure. For individuals who experience this 10 to 15 times a day, the result can be deadly.

TYPES OF STRESSORS

Categories of stress are as follows: (1) physiochemical stressors from the external environment represented by nature, (2) social stressors triggered by the social environment, (3) biologic stressors from the internal environment, and (4) mental stressors from perceived psychologi emotional, or spiritual states.

Each stressor is closely related and works cause stress conditions in a person. The types stress are interrelated; therefore, interventio need to be considered holistically. In other word strategies must address the body, mind, and spi of the individual. The following factors can contri ute to stress:

- Perception. Individuals react differently stress. One nurse may find a leadersh position in management to be invigorati and fun, whereas another nurse may overwhelmed and end up with heart d ease caused by the constant work stres In addition to the perceived work stre level, evaluation of other perceiv stressors that might affect an individu are important to assess.
- Personality. Personalities vary, and some pe sonality types respond negatively stress. If a nurse leader has this type personality, there are stress manageme techniques which increase the ability cope.
- Home and family situation. For some indiv uals, this is the most stressful area of th lives. Many people do not find solace their homes. They may be having difficu with their spouse, children, parents, other family members. The home life of individual is one of the most important e ments when analyzing their stress levels
- Current events. Stress is not only long te but can be triggered by recent ever These events are not necessarily negat in nature and can include marriage, prom tions, and job changes.

In addition, other factors to determine str levels include the following:

- Length of time under stress. The longer a p son has experienced a stressful situati the greater the potential physical and p chologic problems.
- Frequency of the stress. Stress that is countered on a weekly basis is less t the stress of day-to-day contact. H often the stress is experienced makes a ference both mentally and physiologica
- Degree of stress. If the stress itself is a la event, such as a termination from an portant position, stress at very high lev over a relatively short time span is li to occur; however, a smaller amoun stress over a long course of time m

result in the same types of depression and physiologic concerns seen after an extremely large stressful life event. Stress is produced by normal and unusual events as well as by positive and negative occurrences. Just as a divorce or a low-grade event might increase stress, so might positive experiences such as a job promotion or admission to graduate school. Because stress can be cumulative, one needs to monitor and regulate the number of threats (real or perceived), changes, and transitions that are encountered in the same period of time. Stress can be more harmful when one does not feel in control of stress levels and the events that produce them.

SYMPTOMS OF TOO MUCH STRESS

Individuals under stress react mentally and physically. The symptoms of long- and short-term stress are similar and can include the following:

Fatigue
A change in relationship and sociability levels
A change in appetite, either eating more or less
Increased irritability and anxiety levels
An Increase in alcohol, drug, or cigarette use
Body aches and pains not caused by exercise
A change in sleeping or waking patterns
A change in behavior or emotional patterns
An inability to focus on tasks effectively
An inability to concentrate
Depression

Persons are able to tolerate stress in certain amounts and for varying lengths of time. Homeostatic mechanisms afford the body the ability to repair the disturbed systems by absorption of the hormone and chemical surges; however, if the stress level that one is exposed to is too strong for a long time period, the body is unable to adjust properly and symptoms will begin to appear. In these individuals, stress may manifest in an actual physical illness. Treatment of the symptoms may provide short-term relief but is not a long-term solution. Nurse leaders who experience stress need to recognize the symptoms, evaluate the causes, and implement appropriate long-term strategies to reduce stress and transcend it to prevent recurrence.

HOLISTIC APPROACH TO TRANSCENDING STRESS

Nurse leaders in hectic organizational positions are vulnerable to constant stress in the work environment.[9] Such leaders need to understand themselves in body, mind, and spirit to reflect on and realize how the balance of these parts of self exist within them and to determine where they need to focus to rise above (transcend) the stress and rebalance their lives. Once they successfully reflect beyond the circumstances that caused the stress, they are able to develop a more expansive viewpoint and appreciate what is truly meaningful to their lives. Keegan and Dossey[10] define holistic healing as "a process of bringing all parts of one's self together at deep levels of inner knowing, leading toward an integration and balance, with each part having equal importance and value."

Nurses, including nurse leaders, tend to be wounded healers because there is a part in each nurse or nurse leader in need of healing. Nurses and nurse leaders tend to ignore this woundedness by caring for others (at work and outside of work) at the expense of caring for self. As a result, they become exhausted and drained, leaving paths wide open to the body, mind, and spirit for stress to take its toll.[11]

To begin the journey toward stress reduction, rebalance, and transcendence, the nurse leader needs to identify the stressful symptoms starting to manifest themselves, recognize the unhealthy ways he or she is presently dealing with stress, and make a commitment to self-improve. If stress-related symptoms are not yet evident, the goal is to prevent and transcend stress before the onset of symptoms. Nurse leaders who take the initiative to reflect on their stress levels and their behavioral responses to stress in attempt to self-improve will not only help themselves but also act as positive role models for their staff and others with whom they work.

A holistic health perspective to managing stress emphasizes the importance of acquiring a balance between personal and professional lives. It highlights the self-care of the individual as being a critical factor and the importance of being oneself and experiencing oneself to realize the healing needed and to recognize the potentials from within. These thoughts underscore the concept of the wounded healer and propose that individuals must recognize and heal the inner self to allow full attainment of things to which one aspires. The following sections review selected self-care holistic strategies for managing stress which nurse leaders may choose to implement. If practiced on a regular basis, they will help nurse leaders learn to transcend stressful situations by changing and improving the mind-body-spirit balance within, which then flows into an external healing environment outside.

MINDFUL EATING

Nurse leaders are familiar with the importance of healthy eating. Appropriate amounts of protein, carbohydrates, fats, vitamins, and minerals help maintain the body's immune system and homeostatic function. A diet that limits fried and fatty food will make the body stronger and make it easier to cope with stress. Even though nurse leaders know about proper nutrition, they may not always make healthy choices for themselves, especially when under stress at work. As an example, a report may be due by 11:30 AM, and a staffing issue may need to be resolved before lunch. These tasks take longer than anticipated, and the time becomes 1:00 PM, which is scheduled for the monthly budget meeting. The opportunity to relax and eat something healthy does not occur. A mouthful of crackers are eaten on the way to the 1:00 PM meeting. After the meeting, the chaotic pace of the afternoon does not let up. Stress levels can rise if this is a daily occurrence in the workplace. After a tiring day, the nurse leader is hypoglycemic upon arriving home, proceeds to the refrigerator, takes out a container of mint chocolate chip ice cream, and indulges in a large bowl of smooth, cold sugar, and fat before supper! Overindulgence in eating high sugar foods that are low in fiber and nutrients due to physical and emotional fatigue and stress only worsens the stress cycle along with harming the body, mind, and spirit overtime. Chronic imbalances in glucose metabolism increase the risks of heart disease and diabetes.[12,13]

Mindful eating is a healthy strategy for transcending this problem.[14] Mindful eating increases awareness of what is eaten and how it tastes. It is a lifestyle change in which individuals learn to plan regular times to eat (three meals a day), select healthy foods, use their senses to enjoy the taste, aroma, and texture of the food they are consuming, and eat until satiety is produced rather than eating until a feeling of fullness is felt. People are encouraged to slow down and chew their food, take in less food, and better control weight. When nurse leaders learn to enjoy food in the present moment (as it is being consumed), it is a pleasurable experience. They are more likely to make time during work to relax and eat healthy. Nurse leaders who take the time to enjoy a meal and relax are creating a healing environment for themselves that will maintain their health and their effectiveness at work.

EXERCISE AND MOVEMENT

Along with healthy eating, regular exercise has a crucial role in well-being. Physical activity enhances the immune system and helps control obesity, a risk factor for some cancers, heart disease, hypertension, and diabetes. The US Surgeon has increased activity guidelines for adults to include a total of 150 minutes of moderate intensity aerobic activity per week and at least 2 days per week of muscle-strengthening activities.[1] Many activities qualify, such as swimming, bicycling, dancing, housework, and walking. Finding an activity of enjoyment and varying the exercise routine helps to keeps it fresh and fun. The key is to choose a program that meets individual needs and to practice this exercise or activity regularly.

A regular exercise routine can have one of the best influences on reducing physical stress. Exercise can be a short as 10 minutes a day. Long brisk walks can be used after lunch or after a busy day. Other forms of short exercise can be riding a bike to work or parking the car further away from the office and walking the extra distance. Not taking the elevator but walking up the stairs is another exercise easy to fit in a busy day. The more stress is released through brief exercise throughout the day, the more tranquil and in control of self the nurse leader is likely to be.

Other health-minded physical activities for dealing with stress include vigorous activities such as swimming, rowing, and aerobics, and more meditative movement activities such as tai chi, yoga, and qigong. Nurse leaders who have not been practicing vigorous exercise routines may not wish to begin with strenuous activity. Also, it would be important to begin any forceful exercises slowly and to build up at a safe pace that is comfortable and healthy. Depending on the nurse leader's self-assessment, it might be appropriate to seek the approval of his or her primary health care provider first. On the other hand, meditative movement activities are a wonderful way to increase activity that focuses not only on the balance of the physical body but also emphasizes a meditative and spiritual component of self. People use a variety of alternative strategies to deal with stress. The following story describes the life-changing benefits of one of the meditative practices. In the story that follows, a participant of tai chi for stress reduction explains how it made a difference in her life.[16]

I have been taking T'ai Chi in a class twice a week for six months now. Friday morning, this last week, was the morning we chose to do these multiple forms. This experience of multiple forms in a row, with a period of standing Chi Kung in between, takes me deeper and deeper into the experience that T'ai Chi has to offer. I can feel my body loosen with each successive move and I am more deeply relaxed; my body is more open and quiet and grounded with each passing form.

It is interesting how this T'ai Chi experience takes one deeper into the body, expanding and opening the tissues down to the bone. There is nothing else in my life that produces the same result in my body or for my spirit. If I don't do T'ai Chi for a few days I feel my body as noticeably more stiff and less mobile. It feels like a slow but inexorable contraction of my body, like a net being drawn tighter and tighter around me, restricting my movements. This is all reversed after a session of T'ai Chi; it feels like a nurturing breeze is coursing through my body and the pulse of life which is my heartbeat is moving through every part of my body. You know how a piece of music when played softly with passion will allow you to hang on every note until the last one which lingers in the air and expands the seconds after the actual note has played? Well, T'ai Chi expands that last second that is opened up in the music I described; you can live there, look around at your life from that expanded vista and feel yourself connected to the life around you with more than a surface connection. It is as if you are joined and have a perception of a level of reality that is not ordinary and is touching the pulse of life more directly.

At this level, you know the body and spirit are not separate. But the violence done to our bodies, which we accommodate to on a daily basis, closes our spirits and tightens our bodies and obscures the connection between our bodies, our spirits, and ultimately ourselves.

Our reactions to and our interaction with the events of our life have an effect on us. It seems as if there are more contracting events to interact with than expanding events. And you know we remain contracted after our interactions and this contraction in our body and of our spirit remains and, in fact, grows. Think back to the last time you took a long vacation. Remember how it felt? How loose and open and relaxed you felt? How long did it last when you got back in your daily life? Three days? A week?

Incredible isn't it that our state of being can become so pinched just living our lives. Unless we take the time to get in touch and bring those moments of poetry and freedom back into our bodies and consciousness, we remain contracted. The tissues of our body actually change their shape and shorten causing actual physical constriction. T'ai Chi reverses all that. On a daily basis it has the ability to transport you to that state of being you felt from your vacation and beyond. It provides a path for a return to normal, a return to the natural and balanced and open state that is how we were meant to live, freed from the constricting reactivity we generate in just coping with the events of our lives. I thank God everyday that I found T'ai Chi and have an avenue to undue the life stresses that wreak on my body and spirit. I frankly don't know how people who don't do Yoga or T'ai Chi stand it. I think many things help—reading, art, appreciation of beauty, meditation, and physical exercise. When I measure my experience of these activities against what I feel with T'ai Chi though, I find even these wonderful activities give just part of what I feel with T'ai Chi. To combine all those things—working out physically, poetry, beauty, inspiration and art—into one activity which has such a profound and healthful effect on a person is magnificent.

TOUCH THERAPIES

A variety of touch therapies are becoming popular therapeutic nursing interventions for patients to help with relaxation and energy flow. Nurses have also used these therapies with positive effects of tension release. Nurse leaders might find the use of one of these therapies an excellent way to relax, rebalance, and re-energize. Touch therapy includes both hands-on and hands-off techniques. Examples of hands-on techniques are foot reflexology, massage, and Siatsu in which varying motions and depths of pressure are applied to specific areas and points of the body to induce relaxation and other positive preventive or therapeutic effects such as improving circulation, promoting energy flow, pain relief, or aiding in lymphatic drainage.[17–21] In hands-off therapies, such as therapeutic touch and healing touch, the practitioner moves his or her hands through the energy fields surrounding the individual to affect energy field imbalances.[22–25] Nurse leaders need to avail themselves of opportunities to explore the benefits of touch strategies and reap the healthful benefits they offer.

RELAXATION

Thinking peaceful thoughts helps one to feel relaxed. Relaxation methods allege that individuals cannot simultaneously be relaxed and stressed. When a person is in a deep relaxed state, the responses are the opposite of what occurs during a sympathetic response crisis. Relaxation or meditative practices can positively affect pain, blood pressure, coronary heart disease, chemotherapy-related nausea and vomiting, and tension.[26–31] Some examples of relaxation techniques include the following:

Deep breathing. This method consists of taking deep, slow breaths rather than the shallow, rapid breathing that occurs during times of stress. Physiologically deep breathing helps shut off the danger alarm.

Muscular relaxation. This method may be performed while sitting comfortably in a chair or lying down. Tensing and relaxing various muscle groups can work wonders. A simple muscular relaxation technique is to tense the neck and shoulders, shoulder blades, and forehead and eyes for a few seconds, followed by relaxing them. An immediate feeling of unwinding and ease occurs. This simple exercise can be combined with deep breathing by inhaling while tensing and then exhaling during relaxation of the muscles. More sophisticated versions of these muscular relaxation methods, such as the shower of relaxation and progressive muscle relaxation, are easy to learn and helpful to practice.

Relaxation response meditation. This method is the routine practice of quiet concentration focused on one word that is stated slowly as the individual exhales. Meditation frequency is typically a daily session for approximately 20 minutes.

Nurse leaders might try muscular relaxation and deep breathing or meditation to ascertain their effectiveness in decreasing stress. Such methods are easily learned and can be performed at convenient times during the day or evening. Each technique takes practice to incorporate as part of a daily routine, but the benefits of serenity are well worth the time.

IMAGERY

Imagery has been used effectively in several clinical situations to assist patients in imagining the healing taking place within them,[32] to decrease pain,[33–35] and to reduce stress.[36] Nurse leaders can use the powers of the mind to help reduce stress by imagining themselves in a relaxed state. A quiet comfortable place is needed to concentrate and imagine as the person lets his or her mind take them to this peaceful place.

Imaging begins with imagining a peaceful scene, such as lying on the beach, sailing in a fishing boat on a lake, or unwinding in a cabin nestled in the serenity of the mountains. It can be a real place or an imaginary one. All senses are then invoked as the person imagines being in this peaceful, relaxing place. He or she answers the questions, "What do you see? What sounds are there? What sensations of touch, temperature, or smell do you experience?" The person might imagine and feel the warmth of the sun, the coolness of a breeze, the salt tang of the ocean, or the grit of the sand between the toes.

As the imaging continues, the person enjoys visioning this place, relaxation deepens, and the stress subsides. Imaging works well alone or in combination with music therapy.

MUSIC THERAPY

The therapeutic benefits of listening to music have documented decreases in heart rate, blood pressure, and respirations[37–39] and decreased pain and stress in specific clinical situations.[40] Relaxing music reduces production of the stress-related hormones to induce calmness.[41] Nurse leaders can use music therapy as a complement to other stress reduction interventions. Soothing music helps quiet the mind and allows the individual to become peaceful from within. Alternatively, lively music can be stimulating. Music influences an individual's state of the mind. The resultant psycho-physiologic-emotional response balances the body-mind-spirit.

One manner in which to practice the use of music therapy is to lie comfortably and bathe in the music and let it surround the body and the senses. A convenient time is selected, for example, after work, to assist with the transition of leaving work issues until the following day and increasing the ability to be fully present at home with family and friends. Another time to use music therapy might be at night to quiet the mind before going to sleep. Music therapy can also be used during work. Soft music is played on patient care units in many hospitals. A nurse leader might have music playing in the office to offer relief from stress. Music is a wonderful foundation of healing and stress reduction, effortless to incorporate into daily activities, and readily available.

ART THERAPY

Art is another form of stress relief that nurse leaders might consider. The artistic self can be manifested in endless ways such as drawing, writing, poetry, dancing, sculpting, crafts, and music. Engagement in an artful activity helps one to enjoy, focus, and reconnect with self.[42] As one is involved in creating, the negative energy of stress fades

Edmonston[43] uses doodling to help relieve stress. She calls this form of drawing "open-eyed medication." Initially used while in a physician's waiting room to decrease anxiety, she found it kept her focused and grounded. She subscribes to the importance of caring for the spirit and life within to better deal with stress at work and other life challenges.

A mandala is a form of meditative art of Buddhist tradition. The mandala, from the Sanskrit word meaning "circle" or "center," helps a person to center and focus for meditation. A circular design is used to focus the attention and quiet the mind. Nursing schools are beginning to teach this form of art to undergraduate nurses.[44]

Buddhist Monks make mandalas from tiny grains of sand to form magnificent, colorful, complex designs as they focus on inner peace and harmony; however, one can make a mandala using paper and crayons or colored pencils.[45] Mandalas capture feelings on paper in a thoughtful meditative manner. While making mandalas, individuals often discover the self, grow from the experience, and realize enrichment in their spirituality.[46] Feelings and emotions that arise from stressful thoughts are transformed into creative expressions. This meditative activity can help to melt away the feelings of stress.[47]

AROMATHERAPY

Aromatherapy is gaining popularity for use with patients.[48] When used alone or combined with other relaxation therapies, aromatherapy has been shown to decrease agitation, stress, and anxiety levels in patients[49,50] and nurses,[51,52] yet controversy exists among those who do not believe in its effectiveness other than to lift one's mood.[53] The use of essential oils is not new; however, research is beginning to validate the usefulness of these oils when inhaled or topically applied. For example, lavender is an essential oil that has a calming effect and enhances a sense of well-being.[54] Although more research is needed, nurse leaders might try aromatherapy as an adjunct to other holistic stress reduction strategies, such as when relaxing or listening to soft music.

EMPOWERMENT OF OTHERS

Nurse leaders who are transformational leaders motivate staff to perform with excellence.[55] This humanistic leadership style empowers staff to set and achieve goals. Such leaders create healing environments in which to work; therefore, staff satisfaction is high. Communication is open, and staff opinions are listened to by nurse leaders who are genuine and authentic in an environment where respect of one another is valued. Nursing units with transformational leaders are likely to have reduced stress, high recruitment rates, and high retention rates. The nurse leader's investment in promoting a healing environment in which to work will be less stressful for the nurse leader as well as the staff. Ultimately, a healing environment in the work setting extends into patient areas and improves patient care and healing. Health care facilities that support healing environments for patients are successful when there is active participation of its leaders and staff.[56–58]

PROMOTION OF PRACTITIONER-PRACTITIONER RELATIONSHIPS

Relationship-centered care is a model of care giving in which the foundation for care is based on three types of relationships: patient-practitioner, community-practitioner, and practitioner-practitioner.[59] Relationships and interactions among caregivers are essential in forming therapeutic communications that take place in true caring and healing environments.

Nurse leaders are in an excellent position to support healing environments that advance relationship-centered care. In particular, they can set high level expectations of care among practitioners to ensure that practitioner-practitioner relationships are truly genuine and collaborative. Diverse practitioners need to value one another's roles and work together to plan and provide for patient care and healing. When all practitioners feel valued and respected, stress levels are likely to decline. In turn, nurse leaders can spend less time intervening in volatile practitioner-practitioner conflicts and exert their energies in moving care forward on their units or in their departments.

HUMOR

Humor is a powerful stress reliever.[60–62] It also has many other positive health benefits, such as blood pressure management, boosting of the immune system, and increasing lung capacity. Nurse managers can benefit from the positive effects of humor is various ways. During work, appropriate humor can ease tension in a committee meeting. Humor can be used to enhance the healing environment on a clinical unit by improving morale. A happy staff will tend to have good social and working relationships. Humor can be used by nurses to care for patients by having a humor cart with joke books, puzzles, and games. Nurse leaders can extend this gaiety into their personal lives by watching a funny movie after a demanding day at work or by enjoying dinner with family and friends simply to laugh and have a good time. This activity is a terrific way to unwind. Humor is an effective stress-relieving strategy and is fun.

COUNTER CONDITIONING

Recent developments in behavioral psychology promise the possibility of a new drug-free approach to the problem of stress management. Behavioral psychologists have long treated autonomic responses by counter conditioning anxiety, phobias, and other psychologic conditions that are characterized by increased autonomic arousal.[63–65] The sweaty hands, dry mouth, cold feet, tense muscles, and accelerated heart rate of the fearful flyer or anxious dental patient are familiar physiologic manifestations of the anxiety response. Counter-conditioning procedures not only reduce the subjective experience of what the psychologist calls anxiety or stress but also modify its physiologic manifestations. When the individual learns to reduce his or her anxiety, he or she is also learning to lower blood pressure, slow down the heart rate, reduce the tension in muscles, increase the blood flow to extremities, and control the activity of the autonomic nervous system in other ways.

When it was realized that these behavioral procedures produced physiologic side effects with important implications for physical medicine, attention turned from anxiety to stress from neurosis to psychosomatics. Many, if not all, stress-related and psycho-physiologic disorders involve autonomically innervated organs; consequently, many psychosomatic disorders have been demonstrated to be amenable to stress-reducing behavioral procedures. Biofeedback, hypnosis, deep muscle relaxation, and other methods have been used to treat migraine headaches, muscle spasms, essential hypertension, angina, spastic colon, Raynaud's syndrome, sympathetic reflex dystrophy, and many other physical disorders associated with sustained autonomic arousal.

Stress control took on new importance as studies began to indicate that disease processes such as diabetes, arteriosclerosis, and cardiovascular and other physical disorders might be manifestations, to the point of end organ pathology, of chronic sustained autonomic activity. Other studies suggested the involvement of chronic autonomic arousal with the exhaustion and breakdown of the immunologic response and the production of carcinogenesis. Nurse leaders might find counter conditioning a helpful method to combat stress reduction.

COPING STATEMENTS

Learning how to manage feelings and behaviors takes work and practice. One simple way to get started is to develop "coping statements" to counter upsetting thoughts. Coping statements are somewhat like affirmations but are not necessarily positive ideas. Rather, they are realistic or reality based. Coping statements are usually challenges to specific upsetting thoughts and can be used any time.

Individuals need to teach themselves to stop feeling upset, anxious, worried, depressed, angry, guilty, and ashamed, frustrated, and so on. Coping statements may also be used to change undesired urges or behaviors, such as procrastination, smoking, drinking, or taking drugs as a cue to start the process. Individuals learn to observe what thoughts are running through their minds. Once the offending thoughts have been identified, the individual tries to change them. As this ability to use coping statements becomes more familiar, it can be accomplished by disputing or evaluating thoughts on several levels. The main objective is to change one's thoughts in a way that helps one feel or behave differently and less stressed.

CHANGING ANXIETY TO CONCERN

An on-the-spot way to manage a stressful situation is to learn to change anxiety to concern. Concern allows a nurse leader to become motivated to take care of the real problem at hand. He or she learns to identify and change the upsetting thoughts and emotions that are the immediate and proximate cause of the stressful emotion. For example, a nurse leader may be called into the office of an irate department administer. As the nurse leader takes a seat across from his desk, he rudely yells that one of the staff nurses did not have the proper dressing materials ready for a patient and the physician was very angry that this was no way to run a department, and so on. The nurse leader begins to listen as the administrator drones on but she does not react in fear or shrink back. Instead, she quietly looks into his eyes with concern about how his blood pressure is probably going up dangerously high. As she calmly sits there, his high-pitched voice begins to lower to a normal level and his rapid speech slows down. She continues to sit silently, concerned and quiet. He finally has nothing else to say and ceases speaking. She softly and confidently asks, "Is there anything else?" "Well, no," he replies. He is now ready to have a civil conversation about the issue. What had not been relayed to the administrator by the physician was the fact that, because the particular dressing materials requested had never been used in that department before, they were not routinely in stock. Ultimately, the materials had been obtained but apparently not quickly enough for the physician. By changing her reaction from anxiety to concern, the nurse leader maintained control during the conversation and discovered that there really was no crisis and no need for the potential stressful situation.

FINDING THE RIGHT-FIT NURSE LEADER POSITION

Nurse leaders who transcend stress create healing environments for themselves and for the nursing staff with whom they work; however, there are occasions when an organization is not ready to support leaders to create and maintain healing environments in which to work. The fiscal solvency of the organization takes precedence above all else, and nurse leaders may find themselves unable to keep up with the ever increasing and unrealistic work demands thrust upon them. When a nurse leader's repeated attempts to effect positive changes are continuously met with resistance, it leaves him or her feeling overwhelmed and frustrated. In situations like this, it is appropriate to move on. In the midst of the nursing shortage, it is essential for organizations to support nurse leaders, enabling them to enact their roles effectively. More often, health care organizations are recognizing the importance of supporting their nurse leaders to effect change, be visionaries, and take risks implementing new ideas. If the nurse leader is employed in one of the few organizations in which this type of support is only talked about rather than acted upon, it is time to move to another facility in which the administrative support for nurse leaders is sincere.

A STRESS PARABLE

If one compares people to a "mountain," stress tolerance is the "tree" that grows on the mountain. Stressors are the "rain." When the rain called stressor falls, the trees (stress tolerant) that grow on the mountain (people) will store the rain. If the roots of the trees are not wide and evenly spread, there may be landslides. This landslide is the condition when an individual loses to the stress or when he or she becomes affected by stress-related disease. Trees store rain (the stress condition becomes worse). The amount of how much rain (stress) is stored differs according to the tree's roots. The more evenly the root is spread or more strongly the tree is built, the more it can store rain; however, trees also become weaker or ill, and the amount of rain that the tree can store (stress

capacity) becomes less. Nevertheless, rain (stress) is a necessity to live for the trees. Not enough or too much rain is not good for trees. If there is no stress, people will become useless. Also, if rain is being stored, the tree will release the rain from the leaves and roots. This release is the process of stress coping, which removes useless stress.

SUMMARY

Managing stress is important for nurse leaders in all types of leadership roles. It is imperative that nurse leaders evaluate themselves and make long-term healthy lifestyle changes as needed to transcend the stress of competing demands and to rebalance the body, mind, and spirit. This assessment includes taking account of perceived, real, and potential stressors in personal and professional areas. The selected self-care holistic strategies for managing stress included in this article provide examples of interventions nurse leaders may consider to rebalance the internal and external environments of their lives.

Nurse leaders need to create and support healing environments within and external to themselves in all areas of their lives. Internal and external atmospheres of healing reduce stress and promote serenity for nurse leaders as well as those around them. Healing environments will facilitate their abilities to perform as effective leaders, empower the nursing staff with whom they work, and provide healing and caring environments for patients.

REFERENCES

1. Collins N. Taking a lead on stress: rank and relationship awareness in the NHS. J Nurs Manag 2006;14:310–7.
2. Reitveld S, Everaerd W, Creer T, et al. Stress induced asthma: a review of research and potential mechanisms. Clin Exp Allergy 2000;30(8):1058–66.
3. Steward I. Coronary disease and modern stress. Int J Epidemiol 2002;31:1103–7.
4. Devries M, Wilkerson B. Acta Neuropsychiatrica 2003;15(1):44–53.
5. American Health Consultants. Risk of second heart attack doubles with job stress. Case Management Advisor 2008;19(2):21–3.
6. Couser G. Challenges and opportunities for preventing depression in the workplace: a review of the evidence supporting workplace factors and interventions. J Occup Environ Med 2008;50(4):411–27.
7. Keegan L. Therapies to reduce stress and anxiety. Crit Care Nurs Clin North Am 2003;15:321–7.
8. Baier M. Stress and coping. In: Potter PA, Perry AG, editors. Fundamentals of nursing. 6th edition. St. Louis (MO): Elsevier/Mosby; 2005. p. 596–9.

9. Dixon D. Successfully surviving culture change. Journal of Social Work in Long Term Care 2003; 2(3/4):423–38.

10. Keegan L, Dossey BM. Self-assessments. In: Dossey BM, Keegan L, editors. Holistic nursing: a handbook for practice. 5th edition. Sudbury (MA): Jones and Bartlett; 2009. p. 157.

11. Jackson C. Healing ourselves, healing others. Holist Nurs Pract 2004;18(4):199–210.

12. Bloomgarden ZT. Insulin resistance concepts. Diabetes Care 2007;30(5):1320–6.

13. Liu J, et al. Ten-year risk of cardiovascular incidence related to diabetes, prediabetes, and the metabolic syndrome. Am Heart J 2007;153(4):552–8.

14. Engstrom D. Mindful eating: an interview with Dr. David Engstrom. Bariatric Nursing and Surgical Patient Care 2007;2(4):237–43.

15. Surgeon General. Physical activity and health. Available at: www.cdc.gov/physicalactivity/every one/guidelines/adults.html. Accessed December 2, 2008.

16. A healing story: using t'ai chi for stress reduction. Personal case history story.

17. Long A, Mackay H. The effects of shiatsu: findings from a two-country exploratory study. J Altern Complement Med 2003;9(4):539–47.

18. Boost N. The effectiveness of a 15-minute weekly massage in reducing physical and psychologic stress in nurses. Aust J Adv Nurs 2006;23(4):28–33.

19. Cambron JA. Changes in blood pressure after various forms of therapeutic massage: a preliminary study. J Altern Complement Med 2006;12(1):65–70.

20. Quattrin R, Zanini A, Buchini S, et al. Use of reflexology foot massage to reduce anxiety in hospitalized cancer patients in chemotherapy treatment: methodology and outcomes. J Nurs Manag 2006;14: 96–105.

21. Billhult A, Bergbom I, Stener-Victorin E, et al. Massage relieves nausea in women with breast cancer who are undergoing chemotherapy. J Altern Complement Med 2007;13(1):53–8.

22. Brathovda A. Reiki for self-care of nurses and healthcare providers. Holist Nurs Pract 2006;20(2): 95–101.

23. MacNeil M. Therapeutic touch, pain, and caring: implications for nursing practice. International Journal for Human Caring 2006;10(1):40–8.

24. Movaffaghi Z, Hasanpoor M, Farsi M, et al. Effects of therapeutic touch on blood hemoglobin and hematocrit level. J Holist Nurs 2006;24(1):41–8.

25. Eschiti VS. Healing touch: a low-tech intervention in high-tech settings. Dimens Crit Care Nurs 2007; 26(1):9–14.

26. Tacon AM, McComb J, Caldera Y, et al. Mindfulness meditation, anxiety reduction, and heart disease: a pilot study. Fam Community Health 2003;26(1): 25–33.

27. Carson JW, et al. Loving-kindness meditation for chronic low back pain: results from a pilot trial. J Holist Nurs 2005;23(3):287–309.

28. Cheung BM, et al. Randomized controlled trial QiGong in the treatment of mild essential hypertension. J Hum Hypertens 2005;19(9):697–704.

29. Campos de Carvalho E, Martins FTM, Benedita de Santos C, et al. A pilot study of a relaxation technique for management of nausea and vomiting patients receiving cancer chemotherapy. Can Nur 2007;30(2):163.

30. Andrade SK, Anderson EH. The lived experience a mind-body intervention for people living with H J Assoc Nurses AIDS Care 2008;19(3):192–9.

31. Shapiro SL, Oman D, Thoresen CE, et al. Cultivatin mindfulness: effects on well-being. J Clin Psych 2008;64(7):840–62.

32. Epstein GN, Halper JP, Barrett EAM, et al. A pi study of mind-body changes in adults with asthm who practice mental imagery. Altern Ther Heal Med 2004;10(4):66–71.

33. Menzies V, Taylor AG, Bourguignon C, et al. Effec of guided imagery on outcomes of pain, functio status, and self-efficacy in persons diagnosed w fibromyalgia. The Journal of Alternative and Comp mentary Medicine 2006;12(1):23–30.

34. Huth MM, Broome ME, Good M. Imagery reduc children's postoperative pain. Pain 2004;110(1, 439–48.

35. Cregin R, Rappaport AS, Montagnino G, et al. I proving pain management for pediatric patie undergoing nonurgent painful procedures. J Health Syst Pharm 2008;65(8):723–7.

36. Osborne K. Guided imagery and massa Massage and Bodywork 2008;23(3):74–83.

37. Aragon D, Farris C, Byers JF, et al. The effects harp music in vascular and thoracic surgical tients. Altern Ther Health Med 2002;8(5):5 56–60.

38. Chafin S, Roy M, Gerin W, et al. Music can facilit blood pressure recovery from stress. Br J Hea Psychol 2004;9:393–403.

39. Chan MF, Wona OC, Chan HL, et al. Effects of mu on patients undergoing a C-clamp procedure a percutaneous coronary interventions. J Adv N 2006;53(6):669–79.

40. Nilsson U. The anxiety and pain-reducing effect music interventions: a systematic review. AOR 2008;87((4):780–807.

41. Wahbeh H, Calabrese C, Zwickey H, et al. Bina beat technology in humans: a pilot study to ass psychologic and physiologic effects. J Altern C plement Med 2007;13(1):25–32.

42. Repar PA, Patton D. Stress reduction for nu through arts-in-medicine at the university of Mexico hospitals. Holist Nurs Pract 2007;2 182–6.

43. Edmonston C. NTI chapter leadership development workshop speaker manages life's chaos by doodling. AACN News 2007, July;7.

44. Marshall MC. Creative learning: the mandala as teaching exercise. J Nurs Educ 2003;42(11):517–9.

45. Chase T. The wonder of the mandala: circles of wholeness, health, and healing. Int J Hum Caring 2005;9(2):131.

46. Duffy-Randall AT. Mandala: a way of learning transpersonal nursing. Int J Hum Caring 2006;10(3): 57–64.

47. Curry NA, Kasser T. Can coloring mandalas reduce anxiety? Journal of the American Art Therapy Association 2005;22(2):81–5.

48. Buckle J. The role of aromatherapy in nursing care. Nurs Clin North Am 2001;36(1):57–72.

49. Bastard J, Tiran D. Aromatherapy and massage for antenatal anxiety: its effect on the fetus. Complement Ther Clin Pract 2006;12(1):48–54.

50. Perry N, Perry E. Aromatherapy in the management of psychiatric disorders: clinical and neuropharmacological perspectives. CNS Drugs 2006;20(4): 257–80.

51. Cooke M, Holzhauser K, Jones M, et al. The effect of aromatherapy massage with music on the stress and anxiety levels of emergency nurses: comparison between summer and winter. J Clin Nurs 2007; 16(9):1695–703.

52. Pemberson E, Turkin PG. The effect of essential oils on work-related stress in intensive care unit nurses. Holist Nurs Pract 2008;22(2):97–102.

53. Aromatherapy's benefits limited to mood improvement. Harvard Women's Health 2008;15(9):6.

54. Buckle J. Aromatherapy. In: Dossey BM, Keegan L, editors. Holistic nursing: a handbook for practice. 5th edition. Sudbury (MA): Jones and Bartlett; 2009. p. 483–91.

55. Clegg A. Occupational stress in nursing: a review of the literature. J Nurs Manag 2001;9:101–6.

56. Cutshall SM, Fenske LL, Kelly RF, et al. Creation of a healing enhancement program at an academic medical center. Complementary Therapies in Clinical Practice 2007;13:217–23.

57. Blanchet K. The Simms/Mann Health and Wellness Center. Alternative & Complementary Therapies 2007;13(4):207–10.

58. Blanchet K. The Jefferson–Myrna Brind center for integrative medicine. Alternative & Complementary Therapies 2007;13(6):312–7.

59. Koloroutis M, editor. Relationship-based care: a model for transforming practice. Minneapolis (MN): Creative Health Care Management; 2004.

60. Martin RA. Sense of humor and physical health: theoretical issues, recent findings, and future directions. Humor: International Journal of Humor Research 2004;17(1/2):1–19.

61. MacDonald CM. A chuckle a day keeps the doctor away: therapeutic humor and laughter. J Psychosoc Nurs Ment Health Serv 2004;42(3):18–25.

62. Miracle VA. A personal reflection: humor—I'd rather laugh than cry. Dimens Crit Care Nurs 2007;26(6): 241–2.

63. Ward T. Using psychological insights to help people quit smoking. J Adv Nurs 2001;34(6):754–9.

64. Yang PS, Chen CH. Exercise stage and processes of change in patients with chronic obstructive pulmonary disease. J Nurs Res 2005;13(2):97–104.

65. Chung SJ, Hoerr S, Levine R, et al. Processes underlying young women's decisions to eat fruits and vegetables. J Hum Nutr Diet 2006;19:287–98.

Educational Leadership in Professional Nursing

Nancy Girard, PhD, RN, FAAN[a,b,*]

KEYWORDS

- Competencies • History • Leadership • Attributes
- Roles • Outcomes • Education • Curriculum

Nursing educational leadership (EL) has produced the modern nursing profession. The impact has been enormous and permeates every aspect of nursing. EL exists at all levels of education, and nurse educators are transformational agents and leaders who create and direct the constantly changing future of nursing education and practice. Educational leaders function as change agents and leaders to create a preferred future for nursing education and nursing practice. EL requires capacity building at all levels to promote learning and competent, quality performance.

Educational leaders are nursing school deans and associate deans (or top nursing school administrations), department chairs, and faculty. However, anyone involved in education at any level can be an effective and efficient leader of learning. This article discusses EL and the routes to becoming a registered nurse (RN) and the leadership expectations for deans, department chairs, faculty, and staff development educators. Although arguably every nurse is an educator, the focus is on those officially recognized as educational leaders. Additional roles of educational leaders can be curriculum specialists, consultants to schools, accrediting and government agencies, researchers, and international providers of education and development.

Today, EL is more imperative than ever for nursing. Nursing schools are at a breaking point and have not dented the future nursing shortage. The lack of qualified faculty is more concerning than having enough potential students apply to school; it minimizes the potential for future educational leaders. Other concerns with nursing education today include the increase in foreign nurses who have language and cultural differences, an explosion in technologic innovations for health care, and a lack of clinical teaching/practice sites, which forcing educational changes to help manage the health care crises. These factors call for policy changes, reform models, and reform of decades-old curriculum, all of which require leadership to plan, develop, and implement.

HISTORICAL BACKGROUND OF NURSING EDUCATION

Florence Nightingale founded the Nightingale School for Nurses at Saint Thomas's Hospital in London, marking the beginning of professional education in nursing.[1] She introduced a system of recording the sickness and mortality data of the military hospitals. Although she constantly argued that hospitals were not training grounds for nurses but rather on-the-job employment experience, hospitals became the place where nurses trained. (The term *training* still is used today when talking about educating nurses, whether it is a hospital-based school of nursing or a degree granting institution of higher education.) The system did not promote leadership, and the training, although closely monitored, did not contribute to it. Disillusioned with the training of nurses, Florence once said, "I cannot help regretting the present rage for certificates (training completion) and badges. The certificate does not make the nurse, nor does the badge distinguish her as to excellence. Some of our best nurses are without either."[2]

The first schools of nursing were thus hospital-based, causing hospitals to have a tremendous impact on the design and education of nursing. however, this arrangement has not always been ideal. In her attempt to develop a program that

[a] 8910 Buckskin Drive, Boerne, TX 78006-5565, USA
[b] Acute Nursing Care Department, University of Texas Health Science Center, San Antonio, TX, USA
* 8910 Buckskin Drive, Boerne, TX 78006-5565.
E-mail address: ngirard2@satx.rr.com

Perioperative Nursing Clinics 4 (2009) 43–49
doi:10.1016/j.cpen.2008.10.005

women of all socioeconomic levels could attend to gain skills for employment, Florence wanted to improve hospitals by improving hospital nursing and head (matron) nurses. The beginning was rocky, with lectures given by physicians—if they showed up for class—and head nurses who were hostile and often poor managers. The training focus was to prepare cheap workers for the hospital. Hospitals used the nursing students as workforce, and the professionalism desired by Florence did not happen. She felt that theory was separated from practice, and therefore training was fragmented and unplanned. Some nurses became the exceptional ones that Florence envisioned and some, who were without formal training, went on to other hospitals to gain administrative experience. Some leaders opened schools of their own, but the schools remained hospital training centers. EL was then simply role modeling and forging women workers into the sacrificing caregiver that society believed they should be. In 1867, Florence wrote to Mary Jones, superintendent of nurses at St. John's University College Hospital:

> "The whole reform of nursing both at home and abroad has consisted of this. To take all power out of the hands of men and put it into one female trained head and make her responsible for everything regarding the internal management and discipline being performed. Don't let the doctor make himself the Head Nurse and there is no worse matron than the Chaplain."[2]

PRESENT EDUCATIONAL ROADS TO NURSING

Today's hospital-based schools of nursing are the direct descendents of Florence Nightingale's first hospital-based training programs. They were prevalent in the 1950s, gradually declining in numbers as other educational opportunities arose. Some still exist today as originally began, others have joined with community colleges or added a degree program to their exiting one. In the 1950s, most diploma schools had decreased tuition, offering room and board along with education. The student nurses worked in the hospital in addition to learning.

For example, one school in 1958 (Salem City Hospital School of Nursing) charged $300 tuition for the entire 3-year program. In addition to classes, the students worked rotating 8-hour shifts anywhere in the hospital, including delivery and surgical call. No teachers were present and the learning method was "see one, do one, teach one." However, most students felt privileged if they could see a skill first before having to do it;

it was more likely a trial-by-fire situation. [E] primarily involved role modeling and teachin[g] how to work within the hospital system. EL fit th[e] socioeconomic patterns and taught the studen[t] to work hard, fit into the hospital structure, ha[ve] good morals, sacrifice for the good of the patien[t] and obey rules and physicians.

Students were taught the practice preferred [by] the sponsoring hospital, and frequently staye[d] with that hospital throughout their whole care[er]. They learned their lessons well and were excelle[nt] bedside nurses. Graduating students took the [RN] license examination to become RNs. Nurses, a[nd] many of the characteristics of nursing toda[y] remain the same as those taught in diplo[ma] schools. A certificate or diploma was granted [at] the completion of the program. Gradually, as d[e]gree-granting programs increased for nurse[s,] diploma schools were phased out. Only a sm[all] number of these schools remain, or have gro[wn] into a degree-granting program.

Associate degrees (ADs) for nursing are 2-ye[ar] programs given in community colleges. Comm[u]nity colleges serve almost half of the undergrad[u]ate students in the United States, and prepa[re] students for careers or for transfer to 4-year ins[ti]tutions. They graduate approximately 59% of n[ew] nurses today.[3] The nursing programs have pro[lif]erated and equip most nurses to work in terti[ary] care institutions. Graduates can provide excelle[nt] patient care in almost any hospital setting.

Some factors that led to the increase in [AD] programs include the financial ability of [the] students to attend college and the offering [of] a 2-year curriculum, versus 4-year, which enab[les] students to graduate and begin earning mor[e] sooner. Students also take the same RN licen[se] examination as other schools.

The EL leadership with AD programs basic[ally] instills the same goals and ethics as for all nurs[es.] The diploma, AD, and Baccalaureate in Nurs[ing] (BSN) programs provide multiple paths to a nurs[ing] career and remain confusing. The issue of wh[ich] educational program should be entry level divi[des] nursing leaders, and is still unresolved today.

Nurses, usually women, began attending inst[itu]tions of higher learning and, to compete in [the] market place, wanted a degree reflecting t[his] learning. BSN programs are 4 years, with the [first] 2 focused on regular traditional college cours[es] such as history and English. Prerequisite scien[ce] courses are also needed to transfer to nurs[ing]. These first 2 years can be taken in any colle[ge] including a community college, if the courses [are] accepted by another school for transfer. Stude[nts] can then transfer into a university for a BSN deg[ree] or higher.

EL is involved with creating professional nurses that can work in various settings for patient care, and in beginning managerial positions. The National League of Nursing assists in EL by setting standards, guidelines, and assistance. They have developed core competencies for nurse educators, including those for change agent and leader (**Box 1**).

Institutions of higher education offer masters and doctoral degrees for nurses. The Master's of Science in Nursing (MSN) historically has been the degree for specialized advanced nursing practice. Nurses can learn one of four designated advanced practice roles: clinical nurse specialist (CNS), nurse practitioner (NP), midwife, and certified registered nurse anesthetist (CRNA). Nurses obtaining an advanced degree can also major in educational administration, curriculum and instruction, and nursing administration. A new educational major is that of clinical nurse leader. This role envisions the nurse as leader in the health care delivery system across all settings in which health care is delivered, and in education and information management;[4]

Doctoral degrees, as undergraduate degrees, are confusing for both nurses and other health care providers. One can obtain a PhD (research degree), Nursing Doctorate (ND), Doctorate of Nursing Science (DnS), or a Doctorate of Nursing Practice (DNP/Dr.NP).[5]

Some educational leaders recently proposed, amidst much controversy, to have the DNP become the advanced practice degree,[6] and delete the CNS and NP Masters' degree. Concerns were advanced by leaders of the present advanced practice groups, especially CNSs and NPs, that a DNP would not provide any further benefit than the education now offered. They also argue that this move would further fragment nursing education and increase confusion among other health care practitioners as to who can do what, when, and how. Further confusion exists between the roles of the CNS and clinical nurse leader. EL will have to contend with this confusion and bring nursing back into one cohesive body in the future.

EL for nursing education has provided positive and negative outcomes. Nursing has become more visible, recognized, and honored in society. With advanced education, nurses are more equitable to the educational levels of physicians and thus more accepted to work as peers and collaborators. EL has improved patient care safety and promoted wellness in hospitals and the community, and has increased nursing's role from caring for the individual to caring for an aggregate and the community.

However, educational leaders have followed their own paths, sometimes to the detriment to nursing. An example is the extensive fragmentation of nursing education and the increasing ways one can become an RN. The RN licensing examination remains much the same for diploma, AD, and BSN graduates, which hospitals interpret to mean that all RNs are the same, with the same skills and knowledge. The educational routes are confusing for laymen and nurses. Other professions, such as physician, have one way to become a medical doctor (MD), and the level of preparation and what to expect in care are apparent.

The new division, and battle from leaders who do not support the concept, is that of replacing the CNS and NP with a DNP. Advocates state that nurses will then truly be on the same educational and communication level as physicians, and thus will be able to provide better and higher-quality care. Opponents state that hospitals have been very hesitant in the past to hire CNSs at a fair wage, so how can DNPs expect to

---

Box 1

National League of Nursing Core Competencies of Nurse Educators with Task Statements: Competency 5: function as a change agent and leader

Nurse educators function as change agents and leaders to create a preferred future for nursing education and practice. To function effectively as a change agent and leader, the nurse educator:

- Models cultural sensitivity when advocating for change
- Integrates a long-term, innovative, and creative perspective into the nurse educator role
- Participates in interdisciplinary efforts to address health care and educational needs locally, regionally, nationally, or internationally
- Evaluates organizational effectiveness in nursing education
- Implements strategies for organizational change
- Provides leadership in the parent institution as well as in the nursing program to enhance the visibility of nursing and its contributions to the academic community
- Promotes innovative practices in educational environments
- Develops leadership skills to shape and implement change

From National Nursing Staff Development Organization. Core Competencies of Nurse Educators with Task Statements. Available at: http://www.nln.org/profdev/corecompetencies.pdf. Accessed October 9, 2008; with permission.

find a multitude of positions available in a tertiary center. Leaders are trying to guide nursing out of hospitals, into individual and group practice. Moving into the community and out from under hospital rules and regulations and physician control would finally fulfill Florence Nightingale's dream of an autonomous and independent professional nurse.

Although fragmented and convoluted, nursing education still has moved nursing forward. Nursing is considered one of the top professions to enter, and is the most highly respected by laymen. Although curricula in any school remain much the same as they have for 50 years, practice has advanced to keep up with changes in technology and delivery. Nurses have gained recognition and respect with advanced practice roles, have increased the power of nurses in magnet hospitals, and serve as front-line caregivers in both acute care and community settings.

ATTRIBUTES OF EDUCATIONAL LEADERS

EL is more important today than at any time in the past, if nursing is to remain a profession. This practice involves capacity building at all levels, more efficient and equitable ways of providing schooling services, and outcome-based accountability.[7] Thus, new challenges are available for educational leadership, and there is a new focus on content knowledge, learning competencies, and teaching strategies that promote student success in learning. Faculty can now be certified and provide the best practices in curriculum and instruction. The explosion of knowledge is a major challenge for today's educators. In the past, nursing textbooks were slim and brief; students today struggle with 5 lb. books that still must be supplemented with journal research articles. Learning all that is available in 2 years is almost impossible. Thus, the move to a master's degree for entry level is still a viable plan; whether this will evolve in the next decade is yet to be seen.[7]

Educational leaders have identifiable attributes. Specific leadership activity depends on the position and role of the individual. Deans, department chairs, faculty, staff educators, and staff nurses are all educational leaders. Although each individual will serve the needs of the institution, certain attributes of EL will be required.

Deans/Administrators

Dean/administrator is the most common EL role for nursing. Depending on the school or university, the title and the organizational role may differ. Any educational leader must have vision, knowledge, and skills[8–10] to produce desired outcomes. The characteristics of EL at the dean level of administration involve many aspects, including knowledge of the institution and governance and national trends in nursing. Knowledge must also include methods of strategic planning processes and short- and long-term planning tools. These individuals must know the infrastructure and personnel within which they must perform, and the governing board, district, state, and national factors that affect nursing education and curriculum. Strategies to involve and communicate with the community regarding their wellness and health care needs; the ability to raise funding to maintain programs, budget, and marketing; and a comprehensive knowledge of faculty, student, and school needs are important for quality outcomes.

An effective educational leader at this level must work well with the top administrators (eg, university presidents, chief financial officers). Regardless of personal opinion, any public interactions must promote the institution and its leaders in a positive way. A focus on the end goal, bottom line, and results is crucial, rather than details of how to get the goal accomplished. This implies an ability to value opinions and actions of others, and know when and how to delegate work. A leader at this level cannot do it all. He or she must be able to assess a situation quickly and determine if someone else should be doing it and have them do it. If the situation is such that someone else should do it but doesn't know how, they should be taught to do it. The dean should keep only those things for oneself that only the dean can do. Finally, although a dean must be cautious in making promises, all commitments should be kept.

A top leader should have some specific skills, including the ability to clarify, inspire, and guard the shared vision of the organization. Personal skills also include the ability to see the big picture, encourage creative thinking, communicate on all levels, problem solve, make sound decisions, synthesize viewpoints, identify and resolve conflict among faculty and students, and remain positive for the presentation of the future of nursing.

At the top positions, effective educational leadership could have several outcomes, as shown in **Box 2**.

Department Chair

In many schools, the second level of educational leadership is at the department chair level. As with all other roles in nursing and academia, the position may have a different title. In this article, a chair is defined as a leader of a department within the whole of a nursing school. The chair reports to the dean or designee. The department is determined by expertise, such as an acute ca

---

Box 2
Possible outcomes of effective leadership

The nursing school is considered a good place to work and faculty numbers remain consistent

Faculty and students portray a high level of satisfaction

Retention and recruitment is high, student board pass rates are at or close to 100% at all levels,

The budget is in the black and is sufficient to retain optimal numbers of students and viable programs

School passes accreditation at all levels

Graduating students find appropriate jobs immediately

The community is active in school affairs, such as advisory boards, fund raising and promoting the positive image of nursing

There is curricular flexibility to delete nonproductive programs and to begin new ones as the community and societal changes occur

Outstanding faculty teaching, research, and practice are recognized and rewarded

Supports faculty decisions in curricular and scholastic matters

The school, faculty, and students are supported and legally protected

---

department. Programs within a department reflect the expertise, such as medical–surgical nursing, critical care, and perioperative nursing. Faculty with practice expertise, academic credentials, and certification reside within the department. Faculty are hired, evaluated, and mentored by the chair. The leadership role includes administrative, role modeling, knowledge-sharing, and skill abilities.

The chair has knowledge of the vision and plans of the dean and school, and ensures school strategic plans are implemented at a department level. Other specific knowledge includes the relationship of the department budget to school planning, the cost of maintaining faculty and programs, local state and national standards for the specific courses offered, changes in curricular and teaching efforts needed, and the needs of the faculty and students.

Personal characteristics of a department leader can include being a team player and being able to strongly support the dean and higher administration. The department leader must value others and be a good judge of character. The abilities to monitor, guide, evaluate fairly, and terminate

when necessary are essential. As with the dean, the department chair must be able to delegate, honor commitments, and respect faculty, and be able to juggle a myriad of action items at one time.

Skills needed by a department chair are many, and reflect those of a dean. In effect, the chair is running a "mini" school, so the traits are the same. This individual must have a tolerance for ambiguity, because many things in nursing education are not strictly black-and-white facts. The ability to communicate and enunciate values and beliefs is essential. This individual also must have the ability to excel with conflict management and to lead by example and assist faculty to complete department goals and strategic plans. The faculty must be supported in working through the change process. Skills to nurture win/win performances with faculty and identify methods that help students succeed are important to the leadership role.

Fiscal responsibility is paramount, and the chair must be able to develop and manage the department budget. Part of the budget management is the ability to make hard decisions, such as the necessary budgetary abandonment of an educational major that is nonproductive. These decisions must include the skills to design accurate performance indicators to hold everyone accountable for an acceptable workload, and to be able to identify what must be tight versus loose control. Outcomes that reflect positive educational leadership of a department chair are listed in **Box 3**.

Faculty

Individual faculty members are also educational leaders. They must have specific knowledge of their chosen area of practice. This includes the educational requirements, and the appropriate certification. Those involved in research will impact nursing according to their ability to obtain funding, disseminate results of their studies, and work with the community to translate findings into practice. Faculty members must know the content of their courses, and the local, state, and national standards and guidelines. For example, a faculty person teaching perioperative nursing must know Association of PeriOperative Registered Nurses' standards and recommended practices, state nurse practice act requirements, and accreditation needs for their program. Faculty must know theories of teaching/learning and aspects of pedagogy and andragogy to effectively teach the complicated content nursing demands.

Skills necessary for a faculty nursing leader include the ability to lecture, develop curriculum, teach with technology, counsel, mentor, and

---

Box 3
Outcomes that reflect positive educational leadership of a department chair

A department budget that is correctly planned, implemented, and maintained

Funds were raised by various methods to supplement budget shortage

The school and department strategic plan and department goals were annually met, revised, and summarized

Assignment of faculty is fair with manageable work loads

Courses have consistent positive ratings by students

Pass/failure rate of department courses are acceptable within school parameters

Teaching evaluations by students are reviewed, with faculty counseling and rewards given

Conflicts between faculty and students resolved at a department level

Serves on committees within and outside the school

Works with community health care agencies to ensure graduates fit their needs

Department administration is managed with total quality improvement concepts

Is available at all times for faculty and student concerns and problems

---

Box 4
Outcomes of effective educational leadership of faculty

A fully developed and implemented course

Useable and complete courses designed for distance or online

Teaching strategies of large courses, small courses, and individual teaching are effective and appropriate

Use of learning styles contribute to student understanding and performance

Faculty participates in meetings and effectively leads meetings

Faculty communicates well with students, peers, and supervisor

Faculty shares specialty practice information, case studies, and examples with students

Faculty teaches and models evidence-based practice

Faculty effectively evaluates and counsels students

---

communicate with a culturally diverse student body. In addition to teaching skills, faculty members must also excel in clinical practice, be cognizant of the host hospital or health care institution's policies, and be an effective diplomat with the staff of the institution. Outcomes of effective educational leadership of faculty are listed in **Box 4**.

Staff Development Educators

EL in the role of staff educator also occurs, although not as visibly as in academia. These educators have a narrower role and assist nurses working in an institution to maintain competencies, professionalism, and required standards. They uphold the art and science of nursing and promote the image of professional development of the staff. Their leadership role includes encouragement and support of nursing research and the application to practice.[11]

Required leadership knowledge of a staff development educator includes visions and plans for management in health care delivery; strategic planning and fiscal responsibility of nursing;

efficient use of resources; ability to evaluate people, products, and outcomes of care; and teaching/learning needs of the staff. Best safe nursing practices, evidence-based care, and quality improvement theories and methods are vital. With today's reimbursement requirements, the educators must have knowledge of the type of hospital-acquired complications, such as surgical infections, pressure sores, pneumonia, and cystitis. The leadership of the staff educator may become more prominent as care is taught and evaluated to minimize and prevent these nonreimbursable hospital-acquired complications. Although academicians frequently present the best practice and theories gained from research, educational development leaders work in a real-world environment that requires creativity, innovation, and continuous change.

The skills of staff development education leaders reflect those of academic faculty, in addition to their ability to effectively and efficiently work in a bureaucracy of health care. These skills include knowledge of the old and new technology and the ability to use it correctly. They are decision-making educators who must determine when orientation, review, or new information is needed by the staff. Teaching/learning concepts and creatively presenting information to an audience of fast-moving and hard-pressed workers are vital to imparting important information. Finally, they must be able to judge competencies and h

---

Box 5
Successful outcomes of staff educator leaders

Promote consistent compliance with required policies, such as fire control, hand washing, and infection control

Ensure necessary skill levels are present for nursing practice

Ensure new technology is applied and used correctly, and ongoing technology is monitored to ensure continued correct application

Orient all staff to their unit or department

Serve as role model by presenting posters at professional meeting

Contribute to the practice of nursing by writing and presenting quality improvement projects and clinical studies

Maintain certification

Work within a budget

Communicate with community with local conferences or health fairs for professionals and laymen

---

practicing nurses succeed and grow, and appreciate, value, and recognize each person in the organization. Successful outcomes of staff educator leaders are listed in **Box 5**.

SUMMARY

The impact of EL on professional nursing has been enormous and is ongoing. Leaders have forged the present-day nursing profession and continue to change it from within as society's health care needs change. Whether nurses practice at the bedside, in the home, or at a distance, they are functioning because of the molding and shaping provided by educational leaders. The future may prove even more vital as the face and character of nursing continues to evolve and the nursing profession moves toward independent community practice.

Outside the nursing profession, many schools of higher learning have educational opportunities that produce graduate students qualified to be any of the mentioned professionals. University and private schools of nursing offer programs in administration, education, and nursing leadership. These programs can be onsite or given through distance and online methods. An online search enables individuals determine which schools of nursing best fit their career goals. Search terms can be *schools of nursing, online nursing schools,* *accredited schools of nursing,* or *educational leadership.* Specific institutions of higher education can also be reviewed for their offerings. A few examples of accredited schools offering online educational leadership programs are listed in the references.

If one has a desire to attend a college or university onsite to attain a higher degree after graduation from online programs, the institution should be contacted first to see if the credits and degree transfers. Some online institutions offer competency-based learning curricula and a certificate of completion rather than grant a degree.

However one obtains the credentials to be a teacher, EL is a fundamental factor in promoting and advancing the nursing profession. It is present in every situation and aspect and can either be a positive factor or can hinder and delay growth.

REFERENCES

1. Florence Nightingale. (1820–1910). Available at: http://www.morris.umn.edu/~sungurea/introstat/history/w98/Nightingale.html. Accessed 10/9/08.
2. Baly Monica. As Miss Nightingale said... Scutari Press, London; 1991. p. 96.
3. The American Association of Community Colleges. Available at: http://www2.aacc.nche.edu/research/index.htm. Accessed 10/9/08.
4. National League of Nursing NLN CORE COMPETENCIES OF NURSE EDUCATORS 2005. Available at: http://www.nln.org/facultydevelopment/pdf/corecompetenies.pdf. Accessed 10/9/08.
5. American Association of Colleges of Nursing White Paper on the Education and Role of the Clinical Nurse Leader TM, February 2007. Available at: http://www.aacn.nche.edu/Publications/WhitePapers/ClinicalNurseLeader07.pdf. Accessed 10/9/08.
6. Indicators of Quality in Research-Focused Doctoral Programs in Nursing, AACN Position Statement Updated November 2001. Availabe at: http://www.aacn.nche.edu/Publications/positions/qualityindicators.htm. Accessed 10/9/08.
7. AACN. The Essentials of Doctoral Education for Advanced Nursing Practice Available at: http://www.aacn.nche.edu/DNP/pdf/Essentials.pdf. Accessed 10/9/08.
8. Laboratory For Student Success, Delaware MD. Available at: http://www.temple.edu/lss/eduleadership.htm. Accessed 10/9/08.
9. Available at: http://www.aacn.nche.edu/. Accessed 10/9/08.
10. Available at: http://www.nsba.org/sbot/toolkit/Vision.html. Accessed 10/9/08.
11. AACN Position Statement. Updated November 2001. Indicators of Quality in Research-Focused Doctoral Programs in Nursing.

The Advanced Practice Nurse: An Essential Part of the Perioperative Leadership Team

Victoria M. Steelman, PhD, RN, CNOR, FAAN

KEYWORDS

- Advanced practice • Evidence-based practice
- Leadership • Perioperative nursing

The advanced practice nurse (APN) has a vital role in the perioperative leadership team. This person through advanced education coupled with clinical expertise has the background to positively influence the quality of patient care, improve staff safety, and implement evidence-based interdisciplinary changes.

APNs include nurse practitioners, nurse anesthetists, nurse midwives, and clinical nurse specialists. Of these, nurse anesthetists and clinical nurse specialists are found more often in perioperative settings. Nurse anesthetists provide direct patient care to one patient at a time. Clinical nurse specialists are more likely to provide indirect care and be part of the perioperative leadership team. The discussion herein focuses on the leadership role of the clinical nurse specialist.

The American Nurses' Association defines the APN as "The specialist in nursing practice is a nurse who through study and supervised practice at the graduate level (master's or doctorate) has become expert in a defined area of knowledge and practice in a selected clinical area of nursing."[1] In 2004, The American Association of Colleges of Nursing published a position statement advocating for the Doctor of Nursing Practice degree, based on a standardized core curriculum, to be the minimum educational preparation for APNs.[2]

The Association of periOperative Registered Nurses has described perioperative advanced practice nursing and identified different facets of the role as follows:[3]

- Leadership
- Clinical practice
- Education
- Consultation
- Management
- Research

The leadership subrole includes collaboration and coordination with nursing and other disciplines to promote a culture of safety and positive patient outcomes. Clinical practice involves advanced assessment skills, complex physiologic monitoring, and independent judgment. Education is provided for patients, family, personnel, other disciplines, and the public. Consultation is an adjunct to education, providing guidance for the care of individual patients, groups of patients, and a safe environment of care. Management involves defining clinical practice, responding to regulatory requirements, and implementing complex changes. The research subrole involves evidence-based practice and collaborating with others in the conduct of research.

In some perioperative settings, nurse practitioners are being employed to assess patient conditions and prescribe necessary preoperative medication and medical equipment.[4] Nurse practitioners are autonomous, independent, licensed professionals with a scope of practice defined by the state board of nursing. They have prescriptive authority and document in the medical record, including in progress notes and order forms. Within this role, the APN provides care to

Department of Nursing, The University of Iowa Hospitals and Clinics, 200 Hawkins Drive, 6509 JCP, Iowa City, IA 52242, USA

E-mail address: victoria-steelman@uiowa.edu

Perioperative Nursing Clinics 4 (2009) 51–55
doi:10.1016/j.cpen.2008.10.002

individual patients on a patient-to-patient basis. Some nurse practitioners combine advanced practice skills with those of a registered nurse first assistant and provide care to patients preoperatively, intraoperatively, and postoperatively. Clinical nurse specialists, although educated to perform all five subroles described for APNs, are more likely to distribute their workload within one or two of the subroles. They commonly provide indirect patient care and participate as an active member of the perioperative leadership team. This latter role is discussed herein.

THE ADVANCED PRACTICE PERIOPERATIVE NURSE IN A LEADERSHIP ROLE

Individual APNs in leadership positions operationalize their roles differently, dedicating varying percentages of their work time to different subroles. This role division is based on the strengths of the APN and the priorities identified in collaboration with administration in the clinical practice setting. Some APNs focus more on patient care or education, whereas others focus on managerial responsibilities or evidence-based practice.

The subroles are not mutually exclusive, and clinical practice, education, consultation, and management are ways in which the APN demonstrates leadership. The primary objective of the role, regardless of the time distribution between the subroles, is improving the quality of patient care. Leadership through evidence-based practice might be considered a conceptual model to describe advanced practice nursing through which the other subroles are operationalized (**Fig. 1**). In this way, clinical practice, education, consultation, and management are based on the best evidence available, promoting excellence in nursing practice.

CLINICAL PRACTICE AND EDUCATION

Traditionally, perioperative APNs serving as clinical nurse specialists have focused primarily on

the subrole of education. The APN builds upo his or her clinical expertise and understanding the evidence guiding practice to educate ne and existing staff members. Because new grad ate nurses usually have little or no experience the operating room, orientation of new nurs can be labor intensive and comprise a larg percentage of the APN's workload. This work an essential contribution to the leadership tea Orientation offers an opportunity to set the sta for high-quality patient care by teaching best pra tices based on available evidence and instilli a value of inquiry. For example, educating abc risk factors for retained sponges increases comp ance with surgical counts and the attention detail required. Likewise, educating about the ris of perioperative hypothermia increases the like hood that evidence-based measures will be used fectively to promote normothermia. This educati is beyond teaching the actual procedures and e tends to the rationale and evidence to support the practices. It sets the expectation for high-qual care provided within the perioperative setting.

Competency testing is also a part of the educ tion subrole, promoting patient safety by ensuri that staff members are able to perform high ris high volume, or problem prone job responsibilit in a safe manner. Examples of aspects of patie care that an APN may include in competency te ing are listed in **Box 1**.

Competency testing assists the manager w performance appraisal by providing object data about an individual's ability to perform. manager can then design performance impro ment programs for areas of concern.

Ongoing staff development efforts usually foc on safety, including the correct use of new equ ment and changes in established procedur Some examples may include a new fluid warr or ultrasonic dissector. The APN minimizes risk of injury to patients by educating person about how to safely use equipment.

Continuing education programs provide an portunity to teach the rationale for practices more depth, to enhance understanding, and to ther develop the skills of personnel. A course paring nurses for certification is an example of h an APN may develop staff to a higher level of formance than basic competency.

Some APNs provide guest lectures to a demic programs to inspire student nurses to c sider perioperative nursing as a specialty. Oth serve as preceptors, teaching student nurses graduate students. This activity provides an cellent opportunity to role model professic nursing practice and facilitates recruitment nurses.

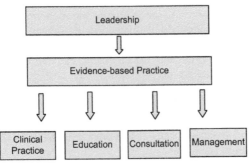

Fig. 1. Leadership in advanced practice nursing through evidence-based practice.

Box 1
Aspects of patient care included in competency testing
Age-specific care
Blood salvage
Care of the morbidly obese patient
Chemotherapy precautions
Definitive care
Documentation
Electrosurgery precautions
Personnel safety
Ergonomics
Prevention of exposures to blood-borne pathogens
Prevention of sharps injuries
Chemical hazards
Smoke evacuation
Laser safety
Latex precautions
Malignant hyperthermia
Pneumatic tourniquet safety
Radiation safety
Sterilization
Surgical counts
Transmissible infection precautions

The perioperative APN may also provide education to patients and family through one-on-one education or by developing educational material. The patient experience in the operating room can be explained better by someone actively involved in patient care. The perioperative APN may work with others to develop a video for preoperative education or written postoperative instructions. Through collaboration with staff members from other patient care areas, programs can be designed to meet the needs of different patient populations and their family members.

The perioperative APN is also called upon to provide outreach education to the public. This education may range from tours of the operating room to presentations to local schools to adult education about perioperative services. In this way, the APN serves as a liaison from the facility to promote health education and the image of the facility.

CONSULTATION

The perioperative APN serves as a resource person to staff members, offering support for complex decision making. Consultations are often made on an individual patient basis or to support decision making for a group of patients. Individual patient consultations include a broad range of clinical issues. Staff nurses often need to make immediate decisions about patient care and have little or no time in which to find and review a policy or search for the best evidence to guide practice. The APN is ideally suited to provide these immediate consultations to maintain the efficiency of the perioperative patient flow while supporting high-quality patient care. Some examples drawn from the log of a perioperative APN are listed in **Box 2**.

These consultations demonstrate the leadership role of the APN in complex decision making as well as providing an opportunity for "just in time" education and mentoring of personnel.

Consultations may also be made to other departments, including anesthesia, labor and delivery, the cardiac catheterization laboratory, interventional radiology, intensive care unit, urology suite, digestive disease suite, preoperative areas, and postoperative areas. These consultations may address infection control, safety, the environment of care, or follow-up on adverse events. With more invasive procedures performed in areas outside of the traditional operating room,

Box 2
Clinical issues addressed by consultation with an APN
Allergy to skin preparation agents
Complex positioning
Dropped cranial bone flap management
Emergency management
Family communication
Forensic evidence management
Incorrect counts
Informed consent issues
Heating, air conditioning, and ventilation issues
Latex allergy
Malignant hyperthermia
Methylmethacrylate precautions
Preoperative fasting
Prevention of hypothermia
Sterilization issues
Supplies opened for extended times
Tissue banking
Transmissible infections
Visitors in the operating room

these extradepartmental consultations are increasingly important for the health care facility. Helping other departments develop policies and procedures for conducting surgical procedures in their areas is one way in which the APN acts as a clinical leader and consultant. Consultations provide an opportunity to collaborate with other departments, ensure the same standard of care for patients undergoing surgery outside of the operating room, and improve patient outcomes.

MANAGEMENT AND PROGRAM DEVELOPMENT

Many perioperative APNs focus a large portion of their workload on managerial responsibilities, including review of standards and regulations, preparation for accreditation surveys, development of new programs or overseeing existing programs, developing policies and procedures, serving on hospital-wide committees, completing short-term projects, and implementing interdisciplinary changes.

During recent years, the number of accreditation or review surveys in health care facilities has increased dramatically. Facilities are seeking overall accreditation (eg, Joint Commission) and for designation as a center of excellence (eg, bariatrics). The Food and Drug Administration surveys tissue banks. Other surveys are performed to determine reimbursement (eg, Centers for Medicare and Medicaid, Occupational Safety and Health Administration) or to investigate patient or staff complaints. The perioperative APN is often called upon to prepare for, coordinate, or respond to survey findings, taking a leadership role in implementing change.

In recent years, more health care facilities are seeking Magnet status through the Magnet Recognition Program, developed by the American Nurses Credentialing Center. This program recognizes health care organizations that provide nursing excellence. Evaluation of the facility is based on quality indicators and standards of nursing practice. APNs are often called upon to provide documentation required to demonstrate that the facility is meeting these quality indicators, or to implement changes to support the Magnet journey.

In addition to accreditation and regulatory compliance, other examples of programs that the perioperative APN may develop, oversee, or dedicate a portion of his or her workload to include bariatrics, conscious sedation, fast track patient care, staff recognition, organ transplants, pain management, quality management, risk management, robotics, skin care, and tissue bank and trauma services.

Managerial projects are usually short term in nature and folded into the workload of the perioperative APN. Examples of managerial projects that an APN may lead include communication and hand offs, continuum of care development, family communication and support, fire safety, national patient safety goals, patient satisfaction, policy revision, product evaluation and product recalls, prevention of wrong site surgery, public relations events, root cause analysis, skin integrity, staff recognition events, and surgeon satisfaction.

In the current rapidly changing health care arena, the managerial role of the APN is also changing. New initiatives provide additional opportunities to make positive changes for patients and personnel.

RESEARCH AND EVIDENCE-BASED PRACTICE

Perhaps the most challenging and rewarding subrole of the perioperative APN is that of evidence-based practice and research. There is increasing demand by professional organizations, accrediting agencies, and consumer groups to base patient care on the best evidence available. To meet this expectation, evidence-based practice might be considered a conceptual framework for advanced practice leadership and integrated into each of the subroles described, including clinical practice, education, consultation, and managerial activities (**Fig. 1**).

The APN may be a leader in the integration of evidence-based changes. One major national evidence-based initiative is the Surgical Care Improvement Project. The Joint Commission, Centers for Medicare and Medicaid, and Institute for Health care Improvement support this collaborative effort to reduce the incidence of surgical complications by 25% by the year 2010.[5] Perioperative APNs are often called up to implement or evaluate compliance with the infection prevention measures (eg, elimination of razor use; appropriate selection, timing, and discontinuation of prophylactic antibiotics) and the targeted interventions to prevent venous thromboembolism. These changes are complex and interdisciplinary. The skills of the APN as a change agent are called upon to maximize the success of implementation of these improvements.

Other evidence-based practice changes may be implemented by the APN in response to new knowledge gained from peer review literature. For example, two chlorhexidine gluconate showers have been found to decolonize patients from *Staphylococcus aureus*.[6] Implementing these preoperative showers has been recommended by the Association of periOperative Registered

Nurses.[7] A second example is implementation of a clinical practice guideline, such as the American Society of Anesthesiologists guidelines for preoperative fasting.[8] Implementation of these changes is complex and requires interdisciplinary collaboration. The APN may serve as the leader in the practice change or a change agent.

APNs also serve as mentors for staff nurses completing evidence-based practice changes. This mentoring extends the work of the APN, implements an opinion leader in the clinical area, and develops the skills of the staff nurse. An example is implementation of an alcohol and chlorhexidine gluconate surgical hand antisepsis. Mentoring a staff nurse to champion this alternative provides the support needed to be successful. Stebral has described an APN-mentored evidence-based practice change to double gloving that resulted in an initial reduction in sharps injuries by 23.5%.[9]

Other evidence-based practice changes are initiated by APNs in response to clinical problems or adverse events. A review of the research on risk factors for retained sponges and instruments identified the need for additional measures to prevent retained objects in morbidly obese patients and major trauma patients undergoing laparotomy. This change required the skills of the APN to present the evidence and influence the opinions of other disciplines and implement a positive change to improve patient safety.

At times, a clinical question arises that requires the conduct of research to answer. This need may best be addressed through a joint effort between the APN and a researcher with advanced education in the conduct of research. The APN may identify the question or work with a staff nurse to articulate the question. Once raised, it may be taken to a researcher, who will need a partner in the clinical setting. This partner may be the APN, who serves as an investigator on the research team. An example is the question "What is the best support surface to prevent intraoperatively acquired pressure ulcers?" APN Cecil King investigated this in collaboration with a researcher.[10] The team found that gel pads are not always the best alternative to disperse intraoperative pressure.

It is essential to base perioperative nursing practice on the best evidence available. The advanced education of the APN supports the questioning of practice, the search for the best evidence available, and implementing complex multidisciplinary changes.

SUMMARY

The APN provides a valuable service to the perioperative leadership team. While managers are busy with day-to-day operations, managing issues with personnel, physicians, and supplies, the APN can focus on long-term objectives such as staff development, clinical decision making, managerial programs and projects, and implementing best practices based on available evidence. This latter contribution will make the APN an indispensable member of the perioperative leadership team in the future. Evidence-based practice can be used as a framework to guide all of the leadership work of an APN. Education should incorporate evidence-based practice. Consultations should include an explanation based on evidence. Managerial programs and projects should be initiated incorporating available evidence. By using evidence-based practice as a framework, the perioperative leadership team can improve patient care and enhance patient outcomes while providing a safe work environment and improving staff satisfaction.

REFERENCES

1. American Nurses Association. Scope and standards of advanced practice registered nursing. Washington (DC): American Nurses Publishing; 1996.
2. American Association of Colleges of Nursing. AACN position statement on the practice doctorate in nursing. October, 2004.
3. Association of Perioperative Registered Nurses. AORN position statement: perioperative advanced practice nurse. Denver (CO): Association of Perioperative Registered Nurses; 2007. p. 403.
4. Guido B. The role of a nurse practitioner in an ambulatory surgery unit. AORN J 2004;79:606–15.
5. Institute for Healthcare Improvement. Surgical Care Improvement Project. 2007.
6. Pottinger JM, Stark SE, Steelman VM. Skin preparation. Periop Nurs Clin 2006;1:203–10.
7. Recommended practices for preoperative patient skin antisepsis. In: AORN, editor. Perioperative standards and recommended practices. 2008 edition. Denver (CO): Association of periOperative Registered Nurses; 2008. p. 537–55.
8. American Society of Anesthesiologists Task Force on Preoperative Fasting. Practice guidelines for preoperative fasting and the use of pharmacologic agents to reduce the risk of pulmonary aspiration: application to healthy adults undergoing elective procedures. Anesthesiology 1999;90:896–905.
9. Stebral LL, Steelman VM. Double gloving for surgical procedures: an evidence-based practice project. Periop Nurs Clin 2006;1:251–60.
10. King C, Bridges E. Comparison of pressure relief properties of operating room surfaces. Periop Nurs Clin 2006;1:261–6.

Implementing Transformational Leadership and Nurse Manager Support Through Coaching

Vicki D. Batson, RN, MSN, CNOR, NEA-BC[a,b,]*,
Linda H. Yoder, RN, MBA, PhD, AOCN, FAAN[c]

KEYWORDS

- Leadership style • Coaching • Transformational leadership
- Work environment • Nurse manager support

The nursing work environment has been the focus of numerous studies over the last decade.[1–6] Elements of a healthy work environment include clear and respectful communication, encouragement of professional practice and support for continued growth and development.[4,7] Leadership practices have been found to either promote or hinder the development of healthy and safe work environments for nurses[3–9] and it is widely recognized that the past two decades of healthcare reform and restructuring had a profoundly negative effect on the nursing work environment.[1–3,6,10,11]

The perceived support provided by nurse managers is a key predictor of nursing job satisfaction in today's work environment.[3–9] Unfortunately, much work still needs to be done to improve nursing satisfaction with nurse manager support. In 2006, Boyle and colleagues[12] reported research findings of job satisfaction by unit type. Perioperative and emergency services nurses reported the lowest overall job satisfaction. Satisfaction with nurse manager support was found to be only moderate in all types of units, with perioperative and emergency services nurses reporting the lowest satisfaction with nurse manager support. In 2007,

Lacey and colleagues[13] reported findings from a study of nursing support, workload, and intent to stay in Magnet, Magnet-aspiring, and non-Magnet hospitals. Although scores on all dimensions were found to be higher in Magnet hospitals than other facilities, nurse manager support was found to have the lowest mean dimension scores in all three hospital types. It was believed that increased span of control by nurse managers and the continuing high number of direct reports contributed most to this problem.

What skills and knowledge are important for nurse managers to develop to improve nurse satisfaction? In studies of the nursing work environment and effective leadership practices, transformational leadership was identified as an effective leadership style to provide psychological empowerment and support of staff, and positive patient outcomes.[6,14,15] One critical skill that clearly demonstrates empowerment and support for staff is the ability to coach others. Coaching involves individual consideration, inspiration, and intellectual stimulation of staff, which are core transformational leadership behaviors. The purpose of this article is to discuss the influence of

[a] Seton Medical Center, 1201 West 38th Street, Austin, TX 787045, USA
[b] The University of Texas at Austin School of Nursing, 1005 Stone Forest Trail, Round Rock, TX 78681, USA
[c] Nursing Administration and Health Care Systems Management, The University of Texas at Austin School of Nursing, 1700 Red River, Austin, TX 78701, USA
* Corresponding author. The University of Texas at Austin School of Nursing, 1005 Stone Forest Trail, Round Rock, TX 78681.
E-mail address: VickiBaston@aol.com (V.D. Batson).

Perioperative Nursing Clinics 4 (2009) 57–67
doi:10.1016/j.cpen.2008.10.004
1556-7931/08/$ — see front matter © 2009 Published by Elsevier Inc.

coaching as a transformational leadership skill and describe an effective process for coaching staff.

The healthcare cost containment pressures of the past two decades have negatively affected the ability of nurse managers to provide the support necessary for a healthy work environment.[2,3,6,10,11] During restructuring efforts to improve efficiency in hospitals and other healthcare organizations, nursing experienced decentralization of nursing leadership positions. The number of nursing leadership opportunities at all levels were decreased and remaining nursing leaders were often expected to increase span of control, which often included areas outside of nursing.[2,11,16] Nurse managers were frequently expected to assume accountability for additional nursing units which may or may not have been similar in patient population and focus to their current units. The increase in workload and number of direct reports for nurse manager was not facilitated by additional resources for the nurse managers such as secretarial support. This resulted in decreased trust of nurse managers by staff nurses, decreased overall job satisfaction, and increased turnover.[2,10,13]

Even Magnet facilities were not immune to these negative consequences. Aiken and colleagues[10] studied the impact of restructuring on 12 of the original Magnet hospitals. Comparison of satisfaction data obtained in 1986 and 1998 demonstrated that nursing satisfaction with managerial support decreased from 90% to 70% and manager accessibility decreased from 89% to 43% during that time.

In spite of these findings, there were positive trends. Research demonstrated that visionary, empowering, and supportive nursing leadership had a powerful effect in reducing the negative effect of restructuring.[3,8] Transformational leadership, and shared decision-making structures such as shared governance were found to provide the organizational and psychological empowerment necessary to develop work environments with higher levels of nursing satisfaction.

The Magnet Recognition Program, developed in 1990 by the American Nurses Credentialing Center, continued to grow and develop, from fewer than 60 hospitals in 2000 to almost 300 today. Although this number represents less than three percent of hospitals, the evidence gained over the past 25 years from research of Magnet hospitals provides a strong blueprint of what comprises a professional practice environment for nurses.[5–7,16–20]

Concern also exists that the ability to retain nursing managers is as critical an issue as the projected nursing shortage.[11,21,22] Recent research linked the influence of emotional intelligence and transformational leadership to the engagement and retention of nurse managers.[11,22] Also, in a study of experienced nurse managers, personal and organizational factors that contributed to the engagement and retention of nurse managers were evaluated. Personal factors included passion and engagement by the nurse manager, and the ability to develop staff and provide recognition of staff. Organizational factors that supported nurse manager engagement and retention were the perception of a strong organizational climate and the presence of organizational empowerment.[3,8,22,2] These factors also were identified as important attributes of nurse manager support and highlight the alignment by both nurse managers and staff as to what is important in a professional work environment.

Kramer and colleagues[23] studied nurse manager support behaviors from the staff perspective. One key finding was that nurse manager supportive behaviors had progressed from traditional management practices to leadership behaviors that focused on building trust, credibility, open communication, and mutual respect. Essential support behaviors identified as desirable included being available, approachable, safe, responsive, providing genuine feedback, and motivating staff to develop self confidence, self reliance, and self-esteem. Both coaching and mentoring of staff were specifically identified as key leadership functions for nurse managers. Transformational leadership behaviors were more frequently described than transactional behaviors, which is consistent with other nursing leadership research.[6,8,14]

ESSENTIAL MANAGEMENT PRACTICES: TRANSFORMATIONAL LEADERSHIP AND SHARED GOVERNANCE

Research has clearly demonstrated that leaders are most effective when there is structure that promotes organizational and psychological empowerment for employees. Shared governance an organizational model frequently used in the nursing work environment to promote staff access to information and support for shared decision making about key issues that affect both direct patient care and the work environment.[15] Shared governance requires leadership behaviors that are more transformational than transactional nature, which supports the findings of Kramer and colleagues,[23] who described essential nurse support behaviors as having more transformational than transactional attributes.

Transformational leadership has been identified as an essential leadership practice to promote both patient and nurse satisfaction.[6,14,15] It also has been described as an essential leadership practice that promotes patient safety by helping balance the tension between efficiency (getting it done) and efficacy (getting it right).[6] Transformational leadership behaviors are part of the full range leadership model developed by Bass and Avolio, which describes leadership behaviors on a continuum from non-leadership to transactional and transformational.[24,25] Transformational leadership comprises four key leadership behaviors. These behaviors are categorized as individualized consideration, intellectual stimulation, inspirational motivation, and idealized influence.

Idealized consideration is demonstrated when the nurse manager takes the time to get to know each individual employee, their preferences, concerns, and ideas. The nurse manager accomplishes this through active listening and encouragement via an open exchange of ideas. The manager promotes self development of the employee through consideration of patient care assignments, and special projects or activities that help the employee grow and develop.

The second behavior, intellectual stimulation, is demonstrated when the nurse manager challenges both individuals and groups of staff members to think through issues and problems for themselves; and supports development of self efficacy. This is accomplished through active listening and reflection by the manager. The nurse manager also may need to create an atmosphere of constructive discontent, challenging staff members to view challenging issues or changes from more than one viewpoint and being comfortable with the tension that is created when significant change initiatives are introduced into the work environment. The manager is responsible for helping staff to re-examine assumptions, revisit problems, and formulate new solutions to complex problems.

The third behavior, inspirational motivation, is demonstrated through the nurse manager's ability to provide a compelling vision of the future that staff members are able to accept and move toward. Ideally, the nurse manager presents an optimistic view of issues and is clear about priorities and goals. Complex and strategic issues are translated into key actions for the department and staff and are communicated effectively in clear and simple language. The outcome is that staff expectations are elevated, and staff members are able to achieve more than they or others expect.

The fourth behavior is idealized influence, which refers to the nurse manager's ability to be a credible role model. Nurse managers are seen as role models when they demonstrate integrity, honesty, and credibility, which creates a sense of trust between them and staff. Nurse managers who demonstrate idealized influence demonstrate ethical behaviors on a consistent basis and are direct, trustworthy, and honest in all interactions. They address issues in a straight forward manner, and recognize and celebrate the accomplishments and contributions of all team members. They are strong advocates for their staff and use their influence for the good of both the department and the organization. Kramer and colleagues[23] described this as "walking the talk."

WHAT IS COACHING?

Although the concept of coaching to improve performance is not new, it is re-emerging as an important aspect of leadership in many disciplines, and on an international scale.[26] The current evidence focuses on coaching as a supportive relationship intended to assist staff with developing skills, talents, self efficacy, and promoting both personal and professional growth.[26–31] Coaching moves beyond traditional management practices of directing, supervising, and controlling, to richer leadership practices of communication, collaboration, empowerment (both organizational and personal) and development, recognizing that people are the most valuable asset in any organization.[27–29]

Coaching, very simply put, is "the art of assisting people to enhance their effectiveness in a way that they feel helped."[27] It involves "collaboration between the manager and employee to achieve increased job knowledge, improved skills, a stronger and more positive relationship, and long term personal and professional growth."[31] Coaching clearly differs from other types of career development such as precepting and mentoring. Precepting is a short-term relationship intended to ensure attainment of facility specific and role-specific knowledge for novice nurses and is generally delegated to another peer who is more clinically competent and has appropriate skills in precepting others. There is a greater focus on task accomplishment and less on the interpersonal aspects of the process.[30,31]

Mentoring is a sustained interpersonal relationship between a senior person with experience, influence, and power who provides information, advice, and emotional support for a junior person, who may or may not be a direct report. The goal of mentoring is to provide specific opportunities for career advancement of the junior person and succession planning for the organization.[30]

While coaching has been used extensively as a basic leadership skill in other disciplines, its consistent use in nursing is not well established. Models for coaching, therefore, are emerging from other professions, most notably business and social psychology. Coaching behaviors are typically measured indirectly as social support and empowerment in nursing research and most recently have been directly identified, as have staff nurse's descriptions of nurse manager support behaviors.[3,8,9,23,26]

Two basic types of coaching have been described in the literature: internal or traditional coaching, and external or executive coaching. The essential difference in the two models is the reporting relationship between the coach and the person being coached and the type of interaction. The internal or traditional coaching model involves an ongoing process of face-to-face interaction between the manager or direct supervisor and employee. This traditional boss–subordinate role does not require that the manager be skilled or credentialed as a coach. However, coaching is most effective when the manager does have the necessary skills and experience, and values having a coaching relationship with the employee. The external or executive coaching model is primarily used for senior- or executive-level leadership development and the coach is neither the direct supervisor of the manager being coached or an employee of the organization. Coaches in this model are frequently external consultants with established credentials as professional coaches. External coaching may be accomplished through a face-to-face interaction or may be done by telephone, email, or video conference. It is believed that the use of external coaches for managers and leaders promotes greater trust in the process and enhances learning and leadership development.[32] Although providing external coaching resources to staff may be cost prohibitive, it is imperative for nurse managers to understand that staff members have the same need for trust and support to develop their potential.

THE COACHING PROCESS

The coaching process involves four essential elements: establishing an effective coaching relationship, feedback and goal setting, monitoring and support of goal completion, and reward and recognition of goal attainment.[26–29] Therefore, effective coaching uses transformational leadership skills. A summary of the relationship between transformational leadership behaviors, essential nurse manager support behaviors, and the coaching process is provided in **Table 1**.

Effective coaching also takes into consideration generational differences. There are four generational cohorts that have been identified in today's work environment. Experiences in family and educational settings have been different for thes[e] four cohorts, and have, as a result, created prefe[r]ences for how each prefers to be coached an[d] motivated by nurse managers.[32–35] The "sile[nt] generation" also referred to as "traditionalist[s]" are employees over the age of 60. This generatio[n] born prior to 1946, most clearly espouses trad[i]tional American values and views the workplac[e] from a traditional lens. They grew up during th[e] Great Depression and World War II and are by n[a]ture conservative, cautious, and hardworkin[g]. They view authority from the traditional values [of] chain of command and are more used to transa[c]tional leadership styles.[32]

"Baby boomers" represent employees born b[e]tween 1945 and 1960 and are the generation wi[th] the largest representation in the workplace cu[r]rently. The first wave of baby boomers will be of r[e]tirement age during the next decade and the effe[ct] of their retirement from the workforce is predict[ed] to significantly contribute to a workforce shorta[ge] of between 400,000 to 800,000 nurses by the ye[ar] 2020.[32] Retention of this generation in the wor[k]place for as long as possible is a critical issue.

"Generation X" or "Gen X" represents e[m]ployees born between 1963 and 1980. Staff fro[m] this generation grew up in homes with two worki[ng] parents and many were raised in single-pare[nt] households. Gen Xers also are referred to as t[he] "latchkey generation" because of this dynam[ic]. They entered the workforce during a period [of] downsizing and restructuring of nursing, and [as] a result, do not have the same level of organiz[a]tional commitment developed in prior generatio[ns]. They are self reliant as a result of these life expe[ri]ences and have a strong desire for balance b[e]tween work and personal life. Additionally, th[ey] grew up in the expanding technology age a[nd] are very comfortable working with complex te[ch]nology and multitasking. Another interesting [dy]namic of this generation is that nursing may [be] a second career for them rather than their ini[tial] choice of profession.[32–35]

"Generation Y" or the "millennial generatio[n]" consists of people born between 1980 and 2[000] who have been raised during a time of commu[ni]cation and technology explosion. Because of r[me]dia access to information, they have a more glo[bal] perspective and are more comfortable with c[ul]tural diversity than traditionalists or baby boom[ers]. Technology has always been a part of their life a[nd] they are comfortable with complex technology a[nd] learning new skills. The millennial generatio[n is] currently the smallest cohort in the nursing wo[rk]force, but is the future of nursing. This genera[tion] is more interested in nursing as an initial car[eer] choice than Gen X and applications to nurs[ing]

Table 1
Relationship of transformational leadership to supportive nurse manager role behaviors and coaching process

Transformational Leadership Attributes	Supportive NM Role Behaviors	Implications for Coaching Process
Individualized consideration: NM gets to know each employee and their individual likes, dislikes, concerns; and uses this as basis for assignments and growth opportunities. The NM promotes development and provides recognition and rewards.	• NM is available, supportive, safe, and responsive. "Asks for input, listens, and follows through, does not betray confidences."[23] • "Gives genuine feedback—cites specific examples, timely manner, does not flatter. Gives positive and negative feedback."[23] • Appreciates quality of care provided by staff and respects employees' personal lives.	• Relationship building is the foundation of the coaching process. The NM cannot successfully coach without having trust and mutual respect. • Feedback is derived from direct observation of behaviors by the nurse manager. Avoid using indirect observations for coaching whenever possible. • Reward and recognition is the fourth essential element of effective coaching.
Idealized influence The NM demonstrates authenticity—there is congruence between word and deed, allowing the NM to be a credible role model. The NM's behavior demonstrates integrity, honesty, and promotes trust and mutual respect.	• "Walks the talk—operationalizes (sic) cultural values so they become the 'norm.' Doesn't just 'talk a good game'; behavior reflects beliefs and values of the unit/organization. Inspires loyalty and commitment to values by leading through example."[23] • "Utilizes constructive conflict resolutions principles; is diplomatic and a good negotiator."[23]	• To be able to influence others, the NM must demonstrate positive regard for all employees and believe in their ability to develop and grow. • The NM behavior must reflect the organization's mission, vision, and values through both works and actions.
Inspirational motivation The NM demonstrates the ability to motivate staff to achieve goals. The NM is articulate and able to communicate very complex issues in a clear and compelling manner. The result is often that individual staff and the entire team can achieve more than expected.	• Encourages goals that are a stretch for staff and supports training for staff through seminars that promote growth. • "Keeps us informed; is a conduit between staff and upper administration. Makes expectations known and clear."[23]	The NM's coaching efforts are direct and help staff link their personal actions to organizational goals. Is clear about the mission, vision, and values of the organization. When providing support for goal development and monitoring support for goal completion, it is important for the NM to help staff recognize how their efforts promote safety, quality, and teamwork.
Intellectual stimulation The NM is able to manage "constructive discontent" to stimulate staff to move beyond old ways of thinking and dealing with issues. The result is that staff develop increased self efficacy in problem solving abilities.	• "Motivates us to develop our self-confidence, self-reliance, and self-esteem."[23] • "Problem-solves with us till we figure it out; leads us in making changes, especially those that are unpalatable; does not micromanage."[23]	Reflective questions and active listening are essential coaching behaviors that help staff sort through issues and develop solutions. The goal of coaching is to increase staff skill in identifying issues from a broader perspective and generate solutions that benefit both the individual and the organization.

Abbreviation: NM, Nurse manager.

programs significantly increased when they entered the workforce.[32]

ESTABLISHING A COACHING RELATIONSHIP

The coaching relationship is an ongoing process that develops over time between a manager and employee. Building trust and understanding between the manager and employee is critical to the success of any work relationship, and is essential for coaching to be effective. Building an interpersonal relationship requires engagement, active listening, and reflection on the part of the manager to ensure that he/she fully understands what matters to employees and what motivates them.[27–29] The process of relationship building initiates the transformational leadership behavior of individualized consideration, provides the manager with greater insight about the employee as an individual, and provides a powerful message of interest and support to the employee. During this phase it also is important for the manager to let the employee know what is important to him/her, both personally and professionally. The nurse manager is responsible for clarifying expectation of performance, and helping employees link their expectations and performance to the organizational mission, vision, values, and goals. This also is the time for the nurse manager to demonstrate by personal behavior that he/she is credible and can be trusted. Staff refer to this by the common term "walking the talk,"[23] which is directly related to the concept of authenticity and the transformational leadership behavior of idealized influence.[24,25]

As the relationship is being established, the nurse manager must establish a feedback loop to ensure that words and behaviors are consistent and convey what he/she is intending to communicate. It is important for nurse managers to understand that in the absence of an established relationship, staff may be uncertain of intent and credibility. Additionally, when there is stress and unpredictability in the work environment, trust may be more challenging to establish.[28] Asking for feedback allows the nurse manager to know when there is confusion or uncertainty, or if intent versus understanding is different. If the nurse manager receives feedback that intent and understanding differ, this provides an opportunity to clarify or apologize and rectify, if appropriate, and to re-establish the foundation for trust building. Without this foundation, coaching will be minimally effective.

Generational differences also influence the successful development of a coaching relationship. Traditionalists expect a clear distinction between the nurse manager and employees, and while they may be on more familiar terms with the nurse manager, when being coached, they are most comfortable with a more professional and official discussion. When developing a relationship with a traditionalist, it is important to remember they are uncomfortable with too much personal information in the workplace. While it is good for the nurse manager to share basic information about personal life, goals, and aspirations, they more quickly relate and appreciate clarity about how their role links to the greater good of the organization, and they are very motivated by the concept of being in service to others.[32,33]

Baby boomers want to make a difference and want to be treated more as equals than subordinates by the nurse manager. Boomers respond well when they feel the nurse manager has truly taken the time to understand them personally and values the unique and individual contributions they bring to the workplace. When establishing relationships with boomers, take time to understand both their work and outside activities. Boomers will be engaged in a variety of outside volunteer activities and also may be responsible for the care of aging parents or grandchildren.[32]

Generation X and Y employees want a very loose relationship with their nurse manager. They want a manager who is very informal, but interested in helping build employees' skills that will serve them over the span of their career. They want support and development, but in a less structured manner than other generations. They value the leadership position, but do not see it as more important than other roles in the unit. Their lack of traditional respect for roles and responsibilities of others with more seniority is often a source of conflict in the workplace. They are easily frustrated by bureaucracy and do not always follow the chain of command for dealing with issues. This is not meant to be disrespectful, but is simply an efficient means of dealing with issues from their perspectives. Visibility and accessibility to this generation are essential behaviors in relationship building as are prompt support for helping them develop skills and experience over time.[32]

FEEDBACK AND GOAL SETTING

Once an effective relationship has been established, the second step of the process, feedback and goal setting, can begin. It is important to remember that the purpose of this step is to create a dialogue that promotes goal setting that is mutually beneficial for the employee and the organization. Initiation of the coaching process is the responsibility of the nurse manager, but there are instances when employees may seek out opportunities both formally and informally about a variety issues. The astute nurse manager is open for these opportunities and makes time for them.[30] Initiation of coaching has been identified by Peterson and Hicks[28] as appropriate in multiple situations. Coaching is most effective when employees actively seek feedback to assist them in career development, but also is necessary when people either do not make development a priority, when they do not know how to learn the skills they need, or when they do not understand their career development needs. Additionally, coaching is needed when people have good intentions, but are not able to translate these into real change in their environment. Coaching is necessary to get employees to believe that you are interested in them and their growth and development.

When initiating the coaching relationship, the responsibility of the nurse manager is to guide the employee through both active and reflective listening to arrive at potential solutions, rather than the manager identifying the issue and proposing a solution. Key to this responsibility, and linked back to the issue of trust, is the ability to demonstrate positive regard for the employee by using direct observation of the employee's skill, knowledge, and behavior as the basis for reflection. Research demonstrates that nurse managers who regard employees as being unable to change or grow coach less often and less effectively.[36]

The nurse manager is accountable for setting an appropriate environment for the coaching interaction—one that is free of disruptions or distractions and is mutually agreeable and convenient to both parties. The nurse manager needs to balance the need for efficiency with the employee's need for a timely discussion. Additionally, the manager should discern if an employee's reluctance to engage in coaching is intended to avoid what may be wrongly perceived as a conflict situation. If coaching must occur to correct or address performance, it needs to happen as soon as reasonably possible to increase effectiveness. If there are other barriers creating a trust issue, the manager should identify and address these barriers to rebalance or re-establish the relationship of trust before proceeding.[28] The agenda or issues to be discussed should be identified beforehand, and each party should be prepared to discuss the issues and focus on generating solutions and actions.

Feedback provided by the nurse manager should be based on direct assessment and measurement whenever possible. Use of third-party feedback should be minimized because it can create miscommunication and trust issues. The most important tool the coach possesses during this interaction is the ability to ask reflective questions that help the employee frame the issue, develop personal insight, and generate actions or solutions that are personally meaningful and can ensure success. Goal setting needs to be mutually beneficial and established in a manner that is satisfying to both the individual and the organization. Identified goals, actions, time frames, and support measures, such as rewards and consequences, need to be fully negotiated and documented. Documentation is powerful as a two-way accountability process for ensuring that both parties commit to their obligations; and it provides a tracking mechanism for monitoring and follow-up.

Initiating a coaching process, providing genuine feedback, and goal setting require new skills for the nurse manager, and require practice and experience to master. Some managers shy away from the process, claiming that it is too time intensive and that they cannot fit it into their busy schedules. However, there are two things that should be considered in response to these objections. The first is that feedback and goal setting are desired and valuable processes for staff and a key indicator of nurse manager support.[23] Although initiation of feedback and goal setting is the responsibility of the nurse manger, once goals are identified, the actions to follow through may be delegated. Additionally, a primary goal of coaching is to develop employee self efficacy, so the need for nurse manager intervention is shifted from doing to supporting. The overall time needed for each coaching encounter will diminish over time with such an investment in the staff. The second consideration is that while learning and becoming comfortable with the process, the nurse manager can choose to start with coaching selected individuals, such as charge nurses and then increase the number of staff coached as coaching skills improve. This also helps to disseminate the coaching process to others who can assist with providing coaching to staff within the unit, especially those nurses on the evening or night shifts.

The initiating process will vary based on the experience and motivational level of the employee; and other variables such as gender, ethnicity, and generational perspectives. The nurse manager benefits from an established relationship with the employee in knowing what level of interaction is required. Traditionalists expect coaching to be initiated as a formal process in the manager's office with no disruptions. When identifying and setting goals, they are more comfortable with a more transactional leadership style, in which the manger provides more direction and less brainstorming or idea generation when formulating solutions to issues.[33] They are most comfortable with a bureaucratic approach where the manager sits behind their desk. To engage employees from this generation in coaching, recognition of their experience and historical knowledge of what has been done before is a good starting point. This demonstrates appreciation of their experience and allows them the opportunity to discuss what has and has not worked in the past. Traditionalists have a strong desire to maintain the status quo. Reflective questions that ask for past experiences dealing with problem are most likely to resonate with this group. Traditionalists prefer discussions to be very straightforward, with clear expectations and information. When setting goals, they prefer to be able to handle one thing at a time, and are not as comfortable with multitasking, computerization, or complex technology. They appreciate being allowed to master new skills, projects, and goals in a linear fashion. They prefer more traditional forms of training such as classroom or lecture presentations by subject matter experts. If learning skills from peers, they need to be matched with a very experienced nurse, and be allowed to learn the concepts before doing them. They do not like to have to learn "on the fly" or in more interactive learning situations such as role playing. Unlike Gen Xers and millennials, they feel foolish and embarrassed when practicing in front of others and prefer to practice skills in a more private manner before having to use them.[32–35]

When initiating coaching with boomers, remember that they want to be treated more as peers than subordinates. In an office setting, they are more comfortable sitting side by side with the nurse manager to have a conversation. Sitting side by side at a table rather than talking over a desk demonstrates willingness by the nurse manager to treat them as equals. Acknowledgement of their personal contributions to the unit is more likely to facilitate engagement in goal setting. A major insight for the nurse manager to keep in mind is that this generation struggles with personal- and work-life balance, related to the conflicts of raising a family, caring for aging parents and possibly grandchildren, and possible commitments to a variety of community volunteer activities. The issue of balance needs to be considered when framing issues and discussing potential solutions. Opportunities for growth and development are always welcome to boomers, who value life-long learning. When gaining new skills they prefer interactive sessions to lectures. They view challenging the "status quo" as their right and duty as a responsible citizen. They value learning strategies that are time-efficient and flexible, such as online learning, or learning advanced skills one-on-one with a more experienced staff member.[32,33]

Initiation of coaching with Gen Xers and millennials requires a more informal approach such as having a soft drink in the office and sitting away from the desk or table. This generation wants know that what they are being asked to do help develop their skill set on a broader basis than the immediate job. This is not intended as disloyalty the organization, rather it is their overall focus f career development. Framing the issues to th larger context of long-term professional develo ment increases engagement. Gen Xers and mille nials prefer negotiations of goals that are fluid terms of means and timeframes. They do n mind being clear about the goals, but want flexib ity in terms of crafting their own strategies to a complish goals. They are self-directed in th learning and are able to use a variety of technol gies efficiently for learning. They prefer experient learning above traditional classroom lectures, a are not afraid of trying new things or role playir They are very willing to learn from another person experiences and are appreciative of a nurse ma ager who is willing to share stories of person shortcomings and learning experiences.[32]

MONITORING AND SUPPORT FOR GOAL ACHIEVEMENT

Once goals are set, the nurse manager's role one of support and encouragement, and monit ing to keep things on track. A vital role for the m ager is to provide reinforcement of progress to t goal over time. The more the goal represe a stretch for the individual, the more the nu manager needs to be available for support and couragement.[28] If the goal builds or rewards talents of a high achiever, the manager's role to be available to ensure there are no barriers goal attainment for the employee.

When monitoring goal attainment by tradition ists, it is important to remember that they acqu skills in a sequential manner and are not comfortable with complex technology. Compu documentation is a troublesome area for this g eration. In the era of electronic medical records is important to remember that some employees this generation may only have traditional typ skills, and they may require more time to mas complex electronic documentation formats. they are struggling to master new skills, enco agement about their importance to the ove unit will help them stay engaged, and they know that their perseverance will be reward Providing additional time and allowing them not feel rushed in mastering new skills also beneficial.[32]

Monitoring progress and supporting boomers is important to ensure that key timeframes are being met. This group may become involved in too many different activities to accomplish each within the desired time frame. Therefore, renegotiation and prioritization of goals may be necessary. The nurse manager should provide encouragement for the individual contribution that is being made by the employee, especially if efforts are part of a larger team, because it is the ability to make an individual impact that is most important to boomers.[33]

Monitoring progress and providing support for Gen Xer and millennial employees presents a special challenge. Support is directed toward removing barriers and allowing these employees to move to the next opportunity as expeditiously as possible. This presents a unique situation in the perioperative setting, where repetition and familiarity of team members enhances safety. The desire of Gen Xers and Millennials to move from service to service once they have learned the basic surgical procedures and their desire to master skills as quickly as possible may create a sense of conflict with traditionalists and boomers, who may believe that each staff nurse or technician needs to "pay dues" and spend longer periods of time before moving to the next service or challenge. The nurse manager will need to help these employees balance between their need for continual learning of new skills and the need to provide stability in work teams. This can be accomplished by working with Gen Xers and millennials to help them understand that spending more time in each specialty can help cement relationships with physicians and other staff that can promote long-term growth.[32] At the same time, the nurse manager must help traditionalists and boomers become comfortable with quicker training and opportunity cycles to help promote retention of younger generations. Allowing Gen Xers and millennials to float between specialty services more frequently can help them keep their skills current in all areas and may provide a sense of support for their growth and development.

REWARDS AND RECOGNITION

Most people want to know that they make a difference and their efforts are appreciated. Saying thank you is one of the most powerful forms of support. Providing ongoing recognition and appreciation to staff facilitates a new cycle of growth and development. Kramer and colleagues[23] found that staff appreciated nurse managers who supported them in decision making and rewarded or recognized exceptional clinical performance. Using the transformational leadership skill of individualized

consideration enables the nurse manager to provide reward or recognition that is personally meaningful to employees. There are many ways to express appreciation and deliberate attention to this aspect of the coaching process is essential.

One creative way that has been reported to provide staff recognition of exceptional clinical achievement is framing and hanging certified perioperative nurse and certified RN first assistant certificates within the department. Departmental newsletters that provide a variety of information also can be used to highlight professional accomplishments of staff members. If monetary awards or paid time off are available within the organization, nurse managers should ensure that their staff has opportunities to receive such recognition. Once again, there are some generational preferences related to this aspect of the coaching process.

Traditionalist value recognition such as handwritten thank-you notes, organizational letters of recognition, plaques or other forms of formal recognition from the nurse manager with a copy sent to their personnel files. Money is still perceived to be the most tangible measure of their work, therefore merit increase for performance or special financial incentives for attaining goals are always powerful expressions of appreciation to them. Flexible staffing that allows them to transition to semi-retirement or relieves them of call responsibilities is valued as a reward for long years of service.[32]

Boomers appreciate public recognition of their achievements and the opportunity to be involved and informed. In addition to traditional recognition, Boomers appreciate the opportunity to participate in special projects or committees or to be funded to outside continuing education activities, especially at a regional or national level. Being given charge or team lead responsibilities also are special forms of recognition and clinical ladder advancement opportunities. Flexible scheduling that allows them to balance work with personal obligations such as elder care and community activities is appreciated.[32,33]

Gen Xers and millennials appreciate traditional recognition and monetary awards, but they also appreciate the next opportunity to learn and grow. They have been described as voracious in their desire to master new skills; offering them special training or learning opportunities is valued as a sign of appreciation for their contributions. They appreciate flexible scheduling as recognition of the value of their personal lives.[32]

RECOMMENDATIONS FOR NURSE MANAGER DEVELOPMENT

Evidence shows that the work environment of nurses is best supported by visible, supportive, visionary, and empowering leadership. Managers who demonstrate transactional leadership behaviors are more effective in engaging the passions and best work of employees. The coaching process purposefully demonstrates nurse manager support behaviors that are desired by employees. Respectful communication, goal setting, support and encouragement of goals, and reward and recognition of achievements truly are elements of a healthy work environment.[4,7,23,27–31] Therefore, managers need to identify their own growth needs and seek coaching for their own skill development. Nurse managers who need additional support to develop coaching skills may seek assistance from more experienced nurses in the organization who have these skills if external coaching is not available. Novice nurse managers also should identify mastering coaching skills as a personal goal when working with their supervisor, who can help them identify resources such as books, journal articles or leadership development conferences to assist them in developing and mastering coaching skills. Many organizations have identified the need to provide leadership development across the organization and continuing education programs or other resources may be available within the healthcare setting. Learning and skill come with practice, and nurse managers can start to build the coaching skill by coaching the charge nurses or informal leaders within the unit or department. This not only allows for skill development, but also helps disseminate coaching skills to these employees who can in turn use them with other employees.

SUMMARY

Coaching is a powerful demonstration of nurse manager support and promotes the development of a healthy and professional practice environment.[23] Coaching uses the transformational leadership behaviors of individualized consideration, idealized influence, intellectual stimulation, and inspirational motivation. These behaviors are used to help develop an effective coaching relationship, set goals, monitor progress, and reward achievements.

Both new and experienced nurse managers need to reflect on the amount of coaching they provide to staff and explore what biases they may have in terms of developing the potential of employees. Seeking feedback about the effectiveness of coaching efforts is important. Research has demonstrated that nurse managers perceive they use transformational leadership behaviors more frequently than employees believe they do.[37] Research also has demonstrated that

managers do not engage in coaching behaviors as frequently if they have a bias that employees are not capable of changing behaviors or improving skills.[38] Therefore, nurse managers need feedback from their employees to ensure they are meeting individual needs for coaching.

Although each employee is a unique individual generational differences between the four generational cohorts that have a direct effect on coaching have been identified. Knowing these differences can assist the nurse manager is using coaching more effectively with these groups. Finally, a primary outcome of coaching is to develop self efficacy of staff. By starting to coach direct reports who have either formal or informal leadership responsibilities, the nurse manager can disseminate a coaching culture within the department a a strategy to foster growth, development, and autonomy at all levels.

REFERENCES

1. Aiken LH, Patrician PA. Measuring organizational traits of hospitals: the revised nursing work index. Nurse Res 2000;49(3):146–63.
2. Aiken L, Clarke S, Sloane D. Hospital restructuring does it adversely affect care and outcomes. J Nur Adm 2000;30(10):457–65.
3. Laschinger H, Finegan J, Shamian J, et al. Impact structural and psychological empowerment on jo strain in nursing work settings. J Nurs Adm 200 31(5):260–72.
4. AACN. AACN standards for establishing an sustaining healthy work environments: a journey excellence. Am J Crit Care 2005;14(3):187–97.
5. Kramer M, Schmalenberg C. Essentials of a magn work environment: part 1. Nursing 2004;34(6):50–
6. Institute of Medicine. Keeping patients safe: tran forming the work environment of nurse. Washingto DC: National Academies Press; 2004.
7. AONE. Principles and elements of a healthful pra tice work environment. Available at: http://ww aone.org/aone/pdf/PrinciplesandElementsHealthf WorkPractice.pdf. Accessed March 21, 2008.
8. Manojlovich M. The effect of nursing leadership hospital nurses' professional practice behavior J Nurs Adm 2005;35(7/8):366–74.
9. Hall D. The relationship between supervisor suppo and registered nurse outcomes in nursing care uni Nurs Adm Q 2007;31(1):68–80.
10. Aiken L, Havens D, Sloan D. The magnet servic recognition program: a comparison of two grou of magnet hospitals. Am J Nurs 2000;100(3):26–3
11. Shirey M, Ebright P, McDaniel A. Sleepless America: nurse managers cope with stress a complexity. J Nurs Adm 2008;38(3):125–31.

12. Boyle D, Miller P, Gajewski B, et al. Unit type differences in RN workgroup satisfaction. West J Nurs Res 2006;28(6):622–40.

13. Lacey S, Cox K, Lorfing K, et al. Nursing support, workload, and intent to stay in magnet, magnet-aspiring, and non-magnet hospitals. J Nurs Adm 2007;37(4):199–205.

14. Wong C, Cummings G. The relationship between nursing leadership and patient outcomes: a systematic review. J Nurs Manag 2007;15:508–21.

15. Batson V. Shared governance in an integrated health care network. AORN J 2004;80(3):494–515.

16. Laschinger H, Wong C, McMahon L, et al. Leader behavior impact on staff nurse empowerment, job tension, and work effectiveness. J Nurs Adm 1999; 29(5):28–39.

17. McClure M, Poulin M, Sovie M, et al. Magnet hospitals: attraction and retention of professional nurses. Kansas City (MO): American Academy of Nursing; 1983.

18. Kramer M, Schmalenberg C. Job satisfaction and retention. Insights for the 90's: part 1. Nursing 1991;21(3):50–5.

19. Kramer M, Schmalenberg C. Magnet hospital nurses describe control over nursing practice. West J Nurs Res 2003;15(4):434–52.

20. Kramer M, Schmalenberg C, Maguire P. Essentials of a magnetic work environment: part 3. Nursing 2004;34(8):44–7.

21. Sherman R. Growing our future nursing leaders. Nurs Adm Q 2005;29(2):125–32.

22. Mackoff B, Triolo P. Why do nurse managers stay? Building a model of engagement. J Nurs Adm 2008;38(3):118–24.

23. Kramer M, Maguire P, Schmalenberg C, et al. Nurse manager support: what is it? Structures and practices that promote it. Nurs Adm Q 2007;31(4):325–40.

24. Kirkbride P. Developing transformational leaders: the full range leadership model in action. Industrial and Commercial Training 2006;38(1):23–32.

25. McGuire E, Kennerly S. Nurse managers as transformational and transactional leaders. Nurs Econ 2006; 24(4):179–85.

26. Stedman M, Nolan T. Coaching: a different approach to the nursing dilemma. Nurs Adm Q 2007;31(1): 43–9.

27. Crane T. The heart of coaching. Using transformational coaching to create a high-performance coaching culture. 3rd edition. San Diego (CA): FTA Press; 2007.

28. Peterson D, Hicks M, editors. Leader as coach—strategies for coaching and developing others. Minneapolis (MN): Personnel Decisions International; 1996.

29. Fournies R, editor. Coaching for improved work performance. New York: McGraw-Hill; 2007.

30. Yoder L. Coaching makes nurses' careers grow. Nurse Week 2007;8(10):24–7.

31. Yoder L. Staff nurses' career development relationships and self-reports of professionalism, job satisfaction, and intent to stay. Nurse Res 1995;44(5): 290–7.

32. Kowalski K, Casper C. The coaching process: an effective tool for professional development. Nurs Adm Q 2007;31(2):171–9.

33. Sherman R. Leading a multigenerational nursing workforce: issues, challenges, and strategies. Online J Issues Nurs 2006;11(2):3.

34. Westin M. Coaching generations in the workplace. Nurs Adm Q 2001;25(2):11–21.

35. Stuenkel D, Cohen J, de la Cuesta K. The multigenerational nursing workforce: essential differences in perception of work environment. J Nurs Adm 2005; 35(6):283–5.

36. Apostolidis B, Polifroni E. Nurse work satisfaction and generational differences. J Nurs Adm 2006; 36(11):506–9.

37. Kleinman C. The relationship between managerial leadership behaviors and staff nurse retention. Research and Perspectives on Healthcare. Hosp Top 2004;82(4):2–9.

38. Heslin P, Vandewalle D, Lantham G. Keen to help? Managers' implicit person theories and their subsequent employee coaching. Personnel Psychology 2006;59:871–902.

Synergy: A Framework for Leadership Development and Transformation

Christine M. Pacini, PhD, RN

KEYWORDS

- Synergy • Leadership development • Orientation
- Professional development • Staff development
- Clinical education

Change in health care as a microcosm of the broader universe is occurring at a rate that makes it almost impossible to keep up. Mechanisms for delivering service, generating relevant products and processes, and reconfiguring systems are becoming increasingly complex. Some of the most formidable characteristics of these systems are that they are inherently uncontrollable and unpredictable, thereby requiring new models and approaches for responsive intervention. For example, such concepts as shared leadership, healing sanctuaries, servant leadership, communities of caring, and self-managed work teams are evolving in support of values related to patient-family centrality, customer-focused behavior, process improvement, safety, and high-quality clinical and behavioral outcomes.

One of the key problems is that past approaches to leading, managing, and learning are far less relevant in environments characterized by values associated with newer knowledge about how change occurs and how individuals think and behave.[1-3] In particular, traditional practices of teaching and learning with regard to aims, content, and methods may now serve as impediments to organizational growth and understanding models of transformation. The content of transformation requires a movement away from industrial, linear thinking toward a focus on integration, outcome, flexibility, responsiveness, holism, contingency thinking, and anticipatory openness to possibility.

The Synergy Model provides a framework for nursing practice and leadership driven by the needs and characteristics of patients, and the predicted demands of the health care environment. The fundamental premise of the model is that patient characteristics drive nurses' competencies. When patients' characteristics and nurses' competencies match and synergize, patients' outcomes are optimized. This paradigm is extraordinarily relevant in that it assumes professional accountability and authority for a clearly articulated set of competencies that vary in light of patient requirements. Moreover, those competencies represent contemporary nursing practice and reflect a dynamic integration of wisdom, experience, values, and knowledge. As such, the model provides a compelling perspective when compared with prior approaches that did not adequately account for the ever-increasing complexities manifested by patients in contexts marked by variability and unpredictability.

This article was originally published in *Critical Care Nursing Clinics* 2005;17(2):113–9.
Center for Professional Development, Research and Innovation, Department of Nursing Services, University of Michigan Health System, 300 N. Ingalls Street, Suite 6819, Ann Arbor, MI 48109-5436, USA
E-mail address: cpacini@Med.Umich.Edu

TRANSFORMING CLINICAL EDUCATION TO SUPPORT LEADERSHIP DEVELOPMENT

As health care and nursing organizations mobilize to design and implement products and processes that demonstrate relevance to the principles and assumptions noted previously, it is apparent that there is a growing dissonance between what is required in the clinical world and what has been incorporated into educational programs. Curricular relevance and integrity are enhanced when faculty and clinical nursing leaders (eg, administrators, managers, clinical educators, advance practice nurses) engage in mutual, ongoing, regularly scheduled, honest discussions about evolving realities and operational standards in practice. In a fully realized, mutual partnership, this dialog rests within legitimate venues of authority and governance; that is, clinical representatives routinely participate in established academic committee venues. Conversely, academic faculty must necessarily partner and participate in similar clinical governance structures.

New paradigms of change should influence processes that impede or delay opportunities for innovation. It is imperative that creativity, applied knowledge, responsiveness, and openness are expected and prevail as normative behavior. As benchmarking related to expected outcomes of clinical performance is the industry standard for measuring organizational value, so must similar constructs of expected, predictable, reliable, and measurable outcomes be applied to educational productivity. Organizations whose means of survival and growth depend on high-quality clinical practice that is tailored and responsive to customers' needs and expectations are increasingly taking on greater responsibility for workforce development. In addition, there is substantive variability in quality and performance of entry-level graduates. It behooves the industry to examine educational outcomes carefully from a perspective that represents the best thinking of both academic faculty and clinical practitioners.

Even assuming that greater educational synergy is accomplished in the near term by implementing enhanced opportunities for interactive dialog between academic and clinical partners, there is always a need for educational intervention in practice settings. The transition from an academic setting to the practice arena is monumental. Pace, volume, and acuity provide the context for new learning and application of principles in real time. Complexity and variability in processes, environment, and personnel further complicate one's trajectory for learning, whether one is new to the profession or new to the organization. Unreasonable expectations for contribution and productivity may add to the "mixture" of risk and insecurity. Growing realization that one has actual authority for a defined scope of practice and is accountable for patient outcomes can provoke a sense of personal distress about limited capacity, or evoke a crisis of trust about others and their level of competency or support. Similarly, clinical managers or directors are charged with patient, environmental, and personnel management while fulfilling new expectations for transformational leadership. In any instance, the implications for learning and development are as complex, variable, and demanding as are the prevailing context and related content.

From the perspective of clinical nursing practice, common implications for educational programming are characterized by the need for breadth, depth, continuity, responsiveness, regulatory sensibility, flexibility, around-the-clock availability, and just-in-time requirements. More importantly, the use of the Synergy Model as an organizing framework propels practice and all related activities toward a sense of mutuality and a shared grasp of foundational principles that drive all professional efforts, the implication being that all "roads" lead to synergy. Whether one engages in direct patient care, serves in a management role, educates staff, or participates in research, the motivation for productivity and evaluation of success is driven by the understanding of patient-nurse centrality. Tenets of the model take into consideration the professional realities of practicing nurses when prescribing performance and role expectations; that is, behavioral characteristics embodying clinical judgment (incorporating wisdom, reasoning, intellectual capacity, and innovation), advocacy and moral agency, caring practice, collaboration, responsiveness to diversity (broadly defined), facilitation of learning, and systems thinking reflect a cadre of competencies essential to meet patient needs. These are not the tenets of ritualistic, task-focused practice or management. Furthermore, patient characteristics are identified and reflect integration about manifestations that drive a professional response. Characteristics of vulnerability, resiliency, stability, complexity, and predictability are not routinely managed from a stimulus-response perspective, nor are they adequately addressed by providers practicing within a hierarchical, maternalistic, or paternalistic scheme of intervention. Rather, the underlying assumption is that patients and families are not bystanders or passive recipients of one-size-fits-all care; they are actively engaged participants in care and decision-making.

Further study and analysis of the Synergy Model reveals opportunities and options for revolutionizing conventional approaches to education in clinical settings. Current practice often focuses on accomplishing regulatory mandates and requirements that may serve to justify the use of methods that have very little to do with clinical or managerial leadership development. Indeed, practice reality requires intervention, documentation, and validation of certain mandates, but is that all there is? In a clinical environment shaped by Synergy, that certainly is not all there is. Synergy is prescriptive for an approach that moves beyond requirement to possibility.

With Synergy, it is no longer acceptable to view a group of newly hired registered nurses as a collection of people conveniently clustered together for the purpose of "giving them what they need." Nurses manifest different strengths and needs with respect to each of the patient and nurse characteristics. Models for learning needs assessment need to be reconfigured in light of nurse attributes conceptualized on a continuum (versus a dichotomous interpretation of competence). For instance, integration of the concept of "safe passage" necessarily implies that the trajectory of orientation, learning, and ongoing development must be shaped by the reality of patient-focused phenomena and outcomes. Differentiated practice and support of professional development requires ongoing competency-based educational programming that facilitates skill development characterized by judgment, intellect, and contribution. Transformational learning experiences require approaches and methods beyond traditional techniques of lecture and demonstration. Experiential learning, which occurs under the guidance of well-prepared clinical coaches or preceptors, facilitates the development of proficiency and expertise.

APPLICATION OF THE SYNERGY MODEL TO CLINICAL NURSING EDUCATION

The journey to educational reformation and transformation can be readily framed or shaped by the Synergy Model. Assumptions about key elements of educational processes and products are derived from and parallel constructs embedded in the model. For example, job documents of registered nurses, clinical managers and directors, educators, and clinical nurse specialists can be configured in terms of the nurse characteristics. Behaviors and criteria for performance evaluation would be described in terms of judgment, advocacy, and collaboration. In addition, clinical, administrative, and educational practices would be differentiated in light of competency, expertise, and contribution. For instance, the Career Advancement Program at Clarian Health Partners and the Professional Development Framework at the University of Michigan

Health System have been implemented to recognize the progression of clinical leadership and differentiated practice for nurses who elect to advance their professional practice while staying at the bedside. These programs identify career levels based on behaviors embedded within the eight nurse characteristics of the Synergy Model (**Box 1**).

Similarly, opportunities for advancement of nursing administrative staff can be constructed by requiring deeper application and use of leadership or managerial principles and competencies. Clinical education roles can be differentiated between those that primarily incorporate tactical or operational responsibilities and those requiring broader application of principles associated with creativity and design, needs assessment, program management, and outcomes analysis (eg, the distinction between an education coordinator and an education specialist). The Role Specific Advancement Model at University of Michigan Health System has been designed to level the progression of practice for education nurse coordinators, clinical care coordinators, practice management coordinators, and flight nurse specialists. Tenets of performance and behavior were derived from the nurse characteristics of the model.

Application of the Synergy Model explicitly implies that educational programming and opportunities for professional development occur in a context of progression, opportunity, choice, competency, and aptitude. Ultimately, patients are the beneficiaries and experience optimal clinical outcomes when their care requirements are matched by the professional competencies of the nurse. Likewise, although more indirectly, the

---

Box 1
Levels of practice

Subsequent to orientation and early development, baseline practice is delineated and describes the work of solidly competent registered nurses with primary responsibilities for patient care. The nurse-to-patient relationship is the primary focus.

As nurses accomplish proficiency in practice, they focus on more complex patients, demonstrate leadership abilities, and contribute to the improvement of patient care at the unit and department level.

As nurses achieve expertise, they may elect to advance to the highest level in either program. These nurses focus on the most complex patients, serve as mentors to others, and contribute to the improvement of their unit or department. In addition, they are expected to contribute on a system-wide level.

same tenet applies when reflecting on the professional development of those in administrative leadership and educational support roles. As competencies of managers and educators are developed in light of transformational principles and evidence, patient outcomes are further enhanced as a consequence of stronger systems leadership and program implementation.

The language and framework of the Synergy Model also provides a useful approach when characterizing learners. The patient characteristics serve as a basis for postulating that learners likely vary across the same dimensions as patients. Mechanisms for assessing learning needs are being reconfigured in recognition of the fact that resiliency, vulnerability, and complexity are detectable manifestations for all kinds of recipients of nursing intervention, including nurses engaged in orientation and other learning programs. It is also hypothesized that use of "ranking" on a continuum (versus dichotomous assessment of task accomplishment) provides more useful baseline data for ongoing developmental planning.

ORIENTATION

Traditional models of orientation customarily provide newly hired employees early on with a substantial volume of required information. Variations on this theme have incorporated Web-based and online validation options, self-study programs, and other approaches for orienting individuals to a wide variety of mandatory requirements. A common view seems to be that there exists a captive audience of learners and a lot of information to "give" them, so the goal becomes to "plow through it all and get it over with." Repeatedly, clinical educators hear: "Well, let's just add that to orientation when they are all together." Any clinical educator or preceptor can easily describe the glassy-eyed look of learners after a week of content saturation and high-volume competency validation.

There is evidence in the literature that many organizations are applying new approaches, content, and methods for evaluating outcomes of these important orientation programs. The concern is that organizations are approaching a level of hypervigilance when it comes to regulatory compliance and mandatory education. Progression toward clinical transformation and fully realized professional practice will not occur if educational resources are stacked so predominantly toward accomplishing these limited, although essential aims. Critical distinctions need to occur in curriculum design from the outset. For example, tenets of educational theory combined with standards for professional development necessarily limit early orientation content

and methods to focus on what is essential and ne essary to know. Attention to patient safety, cue re ognition representing impending crisis and need f support, and resource availability (eg, delegating t to supportive colleagues) provide direction for incl sion and exclusion of relevant content. The impl mentation of orientation should be a tempora organized experience with provision for coordinate interface between didactic and clinical instructic Mutuality and learners' needs must drive teacher i terventions. When there is synergistic interactic learning outcomes are enhanced.

At both Clarian Health Partners and the Unive sity of Michigan Health System, substantive red sign of orientation has been undertaken accomplish the following aims (**Box 2**).

It is clear that this approach to orientation adop a trajectory that is developmental in nature and p ceeds beyond standard time frames for orientatic This does not imply, however, that productivity m gins for individuals are extended beyond reasonak and customary norms. Rather, the model projec a philosophy that "it takes a village" contributing synchrony and harmony to participate in the educ tion of professionals; that it takes time and requir opportunities for experiential learning nurtured other clinical leaders; and that it occurs in a conte of sound educational practice interfaced with re time performance and growth.

ONGOING PROFESSIONAL DEVELOPMENT

The American Nurses Association[4] has outlined scope and standards of practice for nursing profe sional development. Several philosophical sta ments direct one to interpret that the creat work of professional development requires a su stantive commitment far beyond obligations ass ciated with meeting regulatory or task-focus requirements. The work of facilitating the develo ment of fully engaged nursing professionals tr scends a notion of something "nice to do," something essential and necessary. The Syne Model provides an exemplary framework designing and implementing a curriculum that s ports the progression and advancement of nurs in an environment that recognizes and rewards ferentiated practice and clinical leadership. The cus of instruction is to facilitate the enhancemen competencies related to professional contribut and leadership at the unit level. Professionalis transformation, authority and accountability practice, and clinical leadership are the key or nizing constructs for this type of professional nu ing development. Examples of modules that h been implemented at Clarian Health Partners a that fulfill these principles follow.

Box 2
Stages of orientation

Focus early orientation (weeks 1–4) around essential competencies that preserve the safety of patients and use the Synergy Model as an organizing framework for early professional development

Safety and safe passage is the organizing construct for this phase of orientation. Sample content foci include instruction and competency validation for those processes that strongly relate to risk management (eg, legal and regulatory standards and availability and access thereof, nosocomial risk prevention and infection control, cue recognition and processes for "delegating up" when there are questions or uncertainty, communication safety [verbal and written] related to "hand-off" and circumstances of transition, high-volume equipment and process standards [medication administration, fluid management, pump training, patient identification, allergy management, computation validation, and security and confidentiality], and other related content areas).

Support nurses as they apply and implement the model principles in practice (weeks 5–12)

The patient side of the model is the organizing construct for this phase of orientation. Progression in learning moves to more abstract principles and application of existing systems for the purpose of enhancing understanding of the patient and family. Sample content foci include relating existing clinical standards of care and practice to the patient side of the model, discharge planning and developmental approaches to care, family-centered care, palliative and end-of-life care, response to diversity, systems issues and resources related to advocacy and agency, patient-family education, collaboration mechanisms, and opportunities to benefit patients and families.

Provide nursing staff with useful and appropriate developmental tools and opportunities to accomplish performance expectations and meet standards for professional growth and advancement (weeks 12+)

The nurse side of the model is the organizing construct for this phase of orientation. Content foci is developmental in nature and aims to identify short- and long-term options for role development; apply the novice-to-expert framework to one's personal journey of professional development; engage in constructive dialog, communication, and peer feedback; apply principles of leadership to clinical performance; and identify relationships among accountability, autonomy, and clinical outcomes.

Coaching and Effective Communication Skills in the Peer Review Process

This course differentiates between precepting, mentoring, and coaching in regards to definition, purpose, characteristics, and scope. A variety of peer review vignettes are discussed in terms of effectiveness. Strategies for use of constructive feedback in "real world" scenarios are modeled and evaluated with respect to efficacy and potential for accomplishing presumed outcomes.

The Impact of Teamwork, Authority Gradient, and Conflict Management on Patient Safety

This course compares and contrasts characteristics of groups that do and do not function as a team. Importantly, the focus is directed to implications of inadequate team behavior on patient safety and outcomes. Conflict management is discussed from a variety of perspectives (eg, peer-to-peer, patient-nurse, family-nurse, nurse-physician, and nurse-provider). These two initial courses focus on enhancing the learner's communication and negotiation skills within complex patient, family, and staff situations to promote a professional practice environment. Emphasis is placed on improving the learner's abilities to lead a group in consensus building, conflict resolution, and establishing therapeutic relationships within the interdisciplinary team to maximize outcomes for a specific patient population. Honest self-appraisal, independent goal setting, and the desire to reach personal long-term objectives are required.

Evidence-Based Thinking, Data Use, and Tools for Engaging as a Clinical Leader

This course prepares the learner actively to engage in professional accountability for clinical practice at the unit level. Instruction is provided in evidence-based practice and clinical decision-making processes used at unit and system levels. Emphasis is placed on acquainting learners with common practice tools and indicators (eg, report cards, nurse sensitive quality data, and so forth) and their application and use in guiding patient and family-focused clinical practice. This course is designed to address nursing behaviors associated with clinical inquiry and judgment, and responsibility for partner contributions within unit-based shared leadership structures.

Effecting Change in the Practice Environment: Unit as System

This course introduces the learner to two common approaches designed to facilitate the implementation of change in the clinical setting. Components of business planning and project management provide a framework or basis for enhancing skill in the process of collaboration and broadening one's perspective about clinical practice. Change is a fluid and dynamic process and, as such, is facilitated when elements and time frames are clearly delineated within a framework that is understood by those beyond one's immediate purview or setting.

Facilitator of Learning: Taking Accountability Beyond the Bedside

This class is designed to enhance the clinical nurse's ability to assess learning needs, construct objectives or aims to meet learning needs, design and implement teaching strategies to accomplish identified aims, and evaluate the degree to which projected outcomes were accomplished. The course seeks to provide clinical nurses with tools, frameworks, and strategies that position the nurse to work more effectively and broadly with patients, families, and colleagues to facilitate learning. The course is designed to build on fundamental principles of teaching and learning encompassed within the preceptor role or "just-in-time" methods routinely implemented with patients and families.

The Ripple Effect: Caring for People of Many Cultures

This course is designed to provide learners with a basic overview of terminology and concepts related to cultural sensitivity and competence. Concepts are applied in terms of treatment considerations and clinical practice issues. A pretest is included to assist learners in determining their level of self-actualization with respect to this content. Posttesting assesses comprehension and retention of material.

The Code of Ethics for Nurses: a Vehicle for Empowered Caring

This independent study module aims to familiarize nurses with the nine major planks of the current Code of Ethics for Nurses and the accompanying interpretive statements. It orients nurses to the ethical code and how it affects their own nursing practice. It facilitates nurses' ability to use the Code as a guide, and demonstrates how it directs the profession of nursing as a whole. In addition, the module provides nurses with a brief history of the development of the Code of Ethics by the American Nurses Association.

MANAGEMENT DEVELOPMENT

In concert with the aims of embedding principles o leadership within developmental programming fo staff nurses, additional efforts must be imple mented to enhance the ongoing development o managers and directors. Fundamentally, the aim i to study and enhance appreciation for the construc of leadership in terms of new assumptions about th work of administrators and educators. In light o values articulated earlier in the introduction of thi article, redesign of manager orientation and ongo ing administrator development is in process. Again the Synergy Model is useful in providing a frame work for organizing these efforts. The construct o safety and safe passage is primary with respect t manager orientation. Reorganization of content de livery follows a pathway similar to that for sta nurses; that is, administrative knowledge and stan dards of practice related to ensuring patient safet are targeted for instruction early in the orientatio plan. Experienced managers are identified as oper ational coaches. Directors assume responsibility fc evaluating manager progress according to a tem plate outlining competency validation over a perio of approximately 3 months. Similar opportunities fc upward delegation are provided.

SUMMARY

Given the current demands of the health care env ronment, the need for nurses minimally competer in clinical judgment, caring practice, advocac and moral agency, collaboration, responsivenes to diversity, systems thinking, inquiry, and facilita tion of learning is critical in light of ever-increasin contextual complexity and variability of patie needs. The Synergy Model provides an exempla and relevant framework for clinical practice wit the ultimate aim of improving patient outcome Tenets of accountability and professionalism ar central to the model and, in its entirety, it provid a practical and useful approach for thinking abor and redesigning educational products and pr cesses in clinical settings.

REFERENCES

1. Greenleaf RK. On becoming a servant leader. S Francisco (CA): Jossey-Bass; 1996.
2. Goleman D. Working with emotional intelligence. N York: Bantam; 1998.
3. Porter-O'Grady T, Malloch K. Quantum leadersh a textbook of new leadership. Sudbury (MA): Jon and Bartlett; 2003.
4. American Nurses Association. Scope and standar of practice for nursing professional developme Washington, DC: American Nurses Association; 20(

Index

Note: Page numbers of article titles are in **boldface** type.

A

Academic environment, leadership practices for, **1–6**
Accreditation surveys, 54
Administrators as educational leaders, 46
Advanced practice nurse, **51–55**
  definition of, 51
  roles of
    consultation, 53–54
    education, 52–53
    leadership, 52
    management, 54
    program development, 54
    research, 54–55
Antioch University, Center for Creative Change, 4
Anxiety, management of, 38–39
Army Communities of Excellence Program, 4
Aromatherapy, for stress management, 37
Art therapy, for stress management, 36–37
Authority gradient, in professional development, 73
Autonomic arousal, control of, 38–39
Awards, for encouragement, 5

B

Banschbach, Susan K., on enabling others to act, 5
Benner, Pat, Novice to Expert Model of, **23–29**
Body languages variances, 20

C

Challenge the process leadership practice, 3–5
Change, implementing, 73–74
Circular time-orientation perspective, 18
Clarian Health Partners, orientation program of, 72
Clinical research, model for, **23–29**
Coaching, **57–67**
  description of, 59–60
  establishing relationship for, 62
  executive, 60
  feedback in, 62–64
  for professional development, 72–73
  generational considerations in, 60, 62, 64–65
  goal setting in, 62–64
  internal, 60
  monitoring in, 64–65
  process of, 60–62
  rewards and recognition in, 65
  support in, 64–65
  types of, 60

Code of ethics, 74
Communication
  cultural variances in, 19–20
  for professional development, 72–73
  of research findings, 27
Competency, 7, 45, 52
Conflict management, 73
Consultation, advanced practice nurse role in, 53–54
Coping statements, for stress management, 38
Counseling, cultural variances in, 20–21
Counter conditioning, for stress management, 38
Courage, 2
Cultural issues, **17–22**
  allowances of expressiveness, 19–20
  education on, 74
  group-think, 21–22
  paralinguistic variances, 20
  perceptions of time, 18–19
  performance counseling, 20–21
  symbolic interactionism and, 17–18

D

Deans, as educational leaders, 46
Deep breathing, for stress management, 36
Department chair, 46–47
Diet, healthy, 34
Direct work groups, 19
Doodling, for stress management, 37
Duty, 2

E

Eating, healthy, 34
Education
  advanced practice nurse role in, 52–53
  facilitation of, 74
  on politics, 13–14
  Synergy Model applied to, 69–72
Educational leadership, **43–49**
  attributes of, 46–49
  dean/administrator, 46
  department chair, 46–47
  faculty, 47–48
  historical background of, 43–44
  present roads to, 44–46
  staff development, 48–49
Emotions, expression of, 19–20
Empowerment, 8–10, 37
Enable others to act leadership practice, 3, 5

Perioperative Nursing Clinics 4 (2009) 75–77
doi:10.1016/S1556-7931(09)00013-8
1556-7931/09/$ — see front matter © 2009 Elsevier Inc. All rights reserved.

Printed and bound by CPI Group (UK) Ltd, Croydon, CR0 4YY

03/10/2024

01040360-0008